CLINICAL PROTOCOLS
in
OBSTETRICS AND GYNECOLOGY

Dedicated to my mother
and
special thanks to Marti Hudson
who transcribed this book and
is now an expert at flowcharts

PROTOCOLS IN CLINICAL MEDICINE SERIES

CLINICAL PROTOCOLS
in
OBSTETRICS AND GYNECOLOGY

The 'TAN' Book

John E. Turrentine, MD
Hamilton Medical Center, Dalton, GA
Martin Aviles, MD
Hugh Chatham Memorial Hospital, Elkin, NC
and
Joseph S. Novak, MD
Archbold Medical Center, Thomasville, GA

The Parthenon Publishing Group
International Publishers in Medicine, Science & Technology

NEW YORK   LONDON

Published in the USA by
The Parthenon Publishing Group Inc.
One Blue Hill Plaza
PO Box 1564, Pearl River
New York 10965, USA

Published in the UK and Europe by
The Parthenon Publishing Group Limited
Casterton Hall, Carnforth
Lancs. LA6 2LA, UK

First published 2000

Library of Congress Cataloging-in-Publication Data
Clinical protocols in obstetrics and gynecology: the 'TAN' book / edited by
John E. Turrentine, Martin Aviles, Joseph S. Novak.
       p.   cm.
  ISBN 1-85070-308-6 (alk. paper)
   1. Pregnancy—Complications—Handbooks, manuals, etc. 2. Medical
protocols—Handbooks, manuals, etc. 3. Generative organs, Female—
Handbooks, manuals, etc. I. Turrentine, John E. II. Aviles, Martin. III.
Novak, Joseph S.
  [DNLM: 1: Pregnancy Complications—therapy—Handbooks. 2. Genital
Diseases, Female—diagnosis—Handbooks. 3. Genital Diseases,
Female—therapy—Handbooks. 4. Pregnancy Complications—diagnosis—
Handbooks. WQ 39 O137 1999]
RG572.O26 1999
618 21—dc21

                                                99-040821

British Library Cataloguing in Publication Data
  Clinical protocols in obstetrics and gynecology: the 'TAN' book
  1. Obstetrics 2. Gynecology 3. Medical protocols
  I. Turrentine, John E. II. Aviles, Martin III. Novak, Joseph S.
  618
ISBN 1850703086

Typeset by Martin Lister Publishing Services, Carnforth, UK
Printed and bound by Bookcraft (Bath) Ltd., Midsomer Norton, UK

Contents

Introduction

Having been in solo practice for 10 years, I had developed many protocols for the office staff and for myself so that a busy practice could run more smoothly. After all, everyone who works beside a physician likes to be able to predict what he will need for certain procedures or what he will need next for almost anything he does. I had worked with partners for almost 5 years prior to going solo, so I also knew the importance of working together. Knowing how your partner practices his art is important in private practice. There are a hundred ways to 'skin the cat' and practicing medicine is very similar. It is an art and there can be many 'correct' ways to achieve the same goal. However, when several physicians work under the same roof, it is to *everyone's* benefit that they 'grease' the wheels of practice and reach some kind of common goal.

Some physicians, including myself, have had the experience of working with someone who is counter-productive to one's own methodology of practice. One physician gives a patient a prescription or instructs the patient in one manner of practice then 1 week later the patient is back for a follow-up appointment and sees the other doctor. That doctor says, 'Why did he give you that?' He might say, 'That is not the way I do it'. The patient is confused. She is wondering who is right, if anybody. Maybe she thinks she had better reassess her situation. Does this practice know what it is doing? Many patients are lost due to poor communication between staff and doctors or doctors and doctors.

I had the wonderful opportunity to find and work with a real 'dream team' after many years of solo practice. Our team consisted of an experienced and seasoned Ob/Gyn and three well-trained young physicians of different nationalities and sexes. We also had the best nurse that has ever graduated from Emory School of Medicines' Nurse Practitioner Program.

This team was smart, all recently graduated from postgraduate schools and all needed guidance so things would run smoothly. I sat down with the first two new partners in practice and suggested we meet every Friday after lunch to discuss cases and protocols. I thought the protocols would be helpful throughout the remainder of our practice together so we would be on the same team (so to speak).

We began to write a protocol notebook regarding common Ob/Gyn topics, seen both in the office and the hospital. We used ACOG technical bulletins, Ob/Gyn publications, articles, textbooks and computer sources to come up with our own agreed protocol for situations particular for our practice. We tried to develop flowcharts and outlines that would make common problems seem simpler and would be easy to refer to while rushing from room to room during a busy day in the office or hospital. Eventually the notebook was found to be useful to the student doctors, nurse practitioners and other health-care personnel who rotated through the office from nearby North Carolina Baptist and Bowman Gray School of Medicine. Other students from Surry, Emory and Radford University also found the notebook useful and began making copies at the office to help them study. Many suggested that the notebook be published.

I think this book will be useful for any student or practitioner of Ob/Gyn to be able to quickly reference a topic without having to read through thick pages of a textbook to get to the clinical 'meat' of what he or she is looking for. There is certainly room for additional information as the book was written as clinical situations came along during the first year the 'dream team' was together. However, the book has been researched carefully using multiple sources. The protocols are not necessarily the way every Ob/Gyn handles a particular problem. It is the way three Ob/Gyns decided to handle the problems in their office using standard suggestions and recommendations from many reliable sources.

Using the alphabetical table of contents, one can easily find an outline or flowchart on most topics common to Ob/Gyn practice. The topics should certainly be studied from standard textbooks first then the outlines will make much better sense. Nevertheless, this book is meant for quick reference in the office or hospital hall.

Like my first book, *Surgical Transcriptions in Obstetrics and Gynecology*, I hope the '*TAN*' *Book (Clinical Protocols in Obstetrics and Gynecology)* will be useful to those interested in Ob/Gyn care. I certainly enjoyed writing this book with the finest partners a physician could have been associated with. Both Drs Aviles and Novak contributed much of their time and energies to making this book possible. It was certainly more enjoyable being able to share in the ideas for the development of this book rather than work alone. Being faced with many clinical problems, I still reference the manuscript so as to refresh my memory and be certain not to omit an important point or step. I feel that anyone who needs the same quick reference will find this book helpful.

John E. Turrentine, M.D.

ABORTION

DIAGNOSIS AND MANAGEMENT OF RECURRENT PREGNANCY LOSS

Etiology	Diagnostic evaluation	Therapy
Genetic	Karyotype partners	Genetic counseling Donor insemination IVF (*in vitro* fertilization)
Anatomic	Hysterosalpingography (HSG) Laparoscopy Hysteroscopy	Septum resection Cervical cerclage Lyse synechiae Myomectomy IVF, metroplasty, tuboplasty
Endocrinologic	Basal body temperature Endometrial biopsy Mid-luteal progesterone Thyroid stimulating hormone (TSH) Prolactin	Progesterone Clomiphene citrate Thyroid replacement Bromocriptine
Immunologic	APTT VDRL Lupus anticoagulant Antiphospholipid antibiotics	Prednisone Heparin Aspirin
Microbiologic	Cervical culture (*Mycoplasma*, *Ureaplasma*) Endometrial culture	Antibiotics Tetracycline Erythromycin
Metabolic	As indicated	As indicated
Iatrogenic	Tobacco, ethanol abuse Exposure to toxin	Eliminate consumption Eliminate exposure

ABORTION

RECURRENT PREGNANCY LOSS

Name _____

	Normal	Significant results
Genetic		
Karyotype partners	_____	_____
Genetics on POC	_____	_____
Anatomic		
Hysterosalpingography	_____	_____
Laparoscopy	_____	_____
Hysteroscopy	_____	_____
Endocrinologic		
Basal body temperature	_____	_____
Endometrial biopsy	_____	_____
Mid-luteal progesterone	_____	_____
TSH	_____	_____
Prolactin	_____	_____
Immunologic		
Lupus anticoagulant	_____	_____
ANA	_____	_____
Anticardiolipin antibodies	_____	_____
VDRL	_____	_____
APTT	_____	_____
APA	_____	_____
APLA (antiphospholipids)	_____	_____
Infectious		
Mycoplasma hominis	_____	_____
Ureaplasma urealyticim	_____	_____
Toxoplasma gondii	_____	_____
Listeria	_____	_____
Chlamydia	_____	_____
GBBS	_____	_____
Titers for:		
HSV	_____	_____
CMV	_____	_____
Toxoplasmosis	_____	_____
Metabolic		
Panel I	_____	_____
Toxins	_____	_____
Nicotine	_____	_____
Drugs	_____	_____
ETOH	_____	_____

This form may be used in the patient's chart

ABORTION

INCOMPLETE AND/OR RECURRENT

<12 WEEKS

    H&H, WBC, Group & Rh
    Fibrinogen and platelets
    D&E
    D/c 6–8 hrs post-op if stable with minimal bleeding
    F/u 2 wks

13–28 WEEKS

    Offer watchful expectancy at least x3 wks (>4 wks 25–40% DIC) *or* PGE_2; (D&E okay if experienced)
    CBC, fibrinogen, platelets, Group & Rh
    Type & screen
    NPO night before
    Repeat PGE_2 q. 4 hrs
    D5 ½ NS
    Demerol 25 mg IV q. 3 hrs p.r.n.
    Phenergan 25 mg IV q. 4 hrs p.r.n. nausea
    6 hrs post-op – H&H, fibrinogen level
    If USS – d/c x24 hrs – RTO in 2 wks

>28 WEEKS

    CBC w/ platelets, Group and Rh, fibrinogen, Type & cross 2 units; D5 ½
    Pitocin or Cytotech *or* with PG prior to Pitocin
    US q. hr
    Stillbirth protocol (photos, opportunity to view and hold)
    Request autopsy
    Hct & fibrinogen
    If USS – d/c x24 hrs – RTO x2 wks

ABRUPTIO PLACENTAE

DIAGNOSIS

(1) **Clinical symptoms**
Fetal tachycardia/IUFD
Virchow's Triad
uterine pain – focal or generalized
increased tone
vaginal bleeding (85%) – 15% concealed
(2) **Imaging** (ultrasound)
Helpful in concealed abruption – sonolucent retroplacental area
Locate placenta (i.e. r/o previa)

MANAGEMENT

(1) Large bore IV (16 or 18 gauge)
– crystalloid – (LR, D5NS)
– can be used for blood transfusion
(2) Type and cross-match 2–4 units PRBC
(3) Labs: CBC w/ platelets; coagulation profile (fibrinogen, PT, PTT, fibrinogen split products);
repeat q. 2–3 hrs
(4) Continuous EFM, tocometer
(5) Measure serial FH (especially concealed abruption)
(6) Consider central venous access (especially when impending or actual shock suspected)
(7) Strict I&Os (UOP >30 cc/hr)
(8) Determine extent of fetal–maternal hemorrhage (i.e. Kleihauer–Bettke)
Rh neg mother – additional RhoGAM (vial <30 ml)
(9) If stable, spec exam

PLAN

(1) Delivery (when possible)
– low threshold for Cesarean section (fetal/maternal indication)
– if rapid vaginal delivery expected, attempt (or fetus dead)
(2) Expectant management
– patient/fetus stable
– no coagulopathy
(3) Correct coagulopathy
– PRBC
– FFP
– cryo precipitate
– platelets
(4) Correct hypovolemia/restore adequate circulation
– rapid infusion crystalloid/cross-matched blood (O neg in emergency)
– maintain Hct >30%
(5) Avoid incision or episiotomy if possible
– careful hemostasis intrapartum/intra op
(6) Postpartum
– monitor resolution of coagulopathy
– correct anemia, fluid/electrolyte imbalance
– monitor incision/episiotomy site (R/o hematoma)
– strict I&Os

ABRUPTIO PLACENTAE

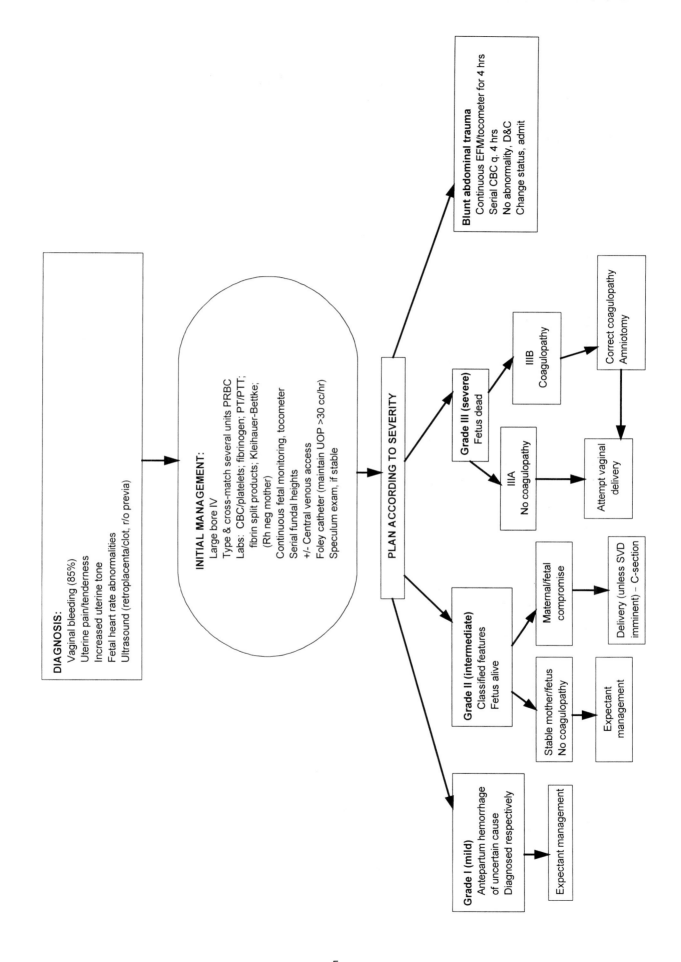

DIAGNOSIS:
Vaginal bleeding (85%)
Uterine pain/tenderness
Increased uterine tone
Fetal heart rate abnormalities
Ultrasound (retroplacenta/clot, r/o previa)

INITIAL MANAGEMENT:
Large bore IV
Type & cross-match several units PRBC
Labs: CBC/platelets; fibrinogen; PT/PTT;
fibrin split products; Kleihauer-Bettke;
(Rh neg mother)
Continuous fetal monitoring, tocometer
Serial fundal heights
+/- Central venous access
Foley catheter (maintain UOP >30 cc/hr)
Speculum exam, if stable

PLAN ACCORDING TO SEVERITY

Blunt abdominal trauma
Continuous EFM/tocometer for 4 hrs
Serial CBC q. 4 hrs
No abnormality, D&C
Change status, admit

Grade III (severe)
Fetus dead

IIIA
No coagulopathy

IIIB
Coagulopathy

Attempt vaginal delivery

Correct coagulopathy
Amniotomy

Grade II (intermediate)
Classified features
Fetus alive

Stable mother/fetus
No coagulopathy

Maternal/fetal compromise

Expectant management

Delivery (unless SVD imminent) – C-section

Grade I (mild)
Antepartum hemorrhage of uncertain cause
Diagnosed respectively

Expectant management

AMBIGUOUS GENITALIA

DEFINITION

Anatomic modification of the external genitalia making specific determination of gender difficult

EVALUATION

The prime diagnosis, until ruled out, is congenital adrenal hyperplasia, because this is the only condition that is life-threatening

DIFFERENTIAL DIAGNOSIS (4 categories)

(1)   Female pseudohermaphroditism
(2)   Male psuedohermaphroditism
(3)   True hermaphroditism
(4)   Gonadal dysgenesis

DIAGNOSTIC WORKUP

(1)   History and physical
      Are gonads palpable? (Most important part of the exam)
      Phallus length and diameter?
      Position of the urethral meatus?
      Degree of labioscrotal fold fusion?
      Is there a vagina, vaginal pouch, or urogenital sinus?
(2)   Pelvic ultrasound or MRI
(3)   Blood for karyotype analysis, serum electrolytes, androgens (androstenedione, testosterone, DHEA, DHEAS), 17-OHP, 11-deoxycorticosterone and 11-deoxycortisol
(4)   In selected cases – laparotomy, gonadal biopsy, and/or gonadectomy; (laparoscopic evaluation is inadequate)

LABORATORY FINDINGS

(1)   Female pseudohermaphroditism (genetic females with excess androgen) in the absence of maternal androgen excess – 3 forms of congenital virilizing adrenal hyperplasia:
      (a)   21-Hydroxylase deficiency – elevated serum 17-OHP
            This is the most common form of congenital adrenal hyperplasia (90%), the most frequent cause of sexual ambiguity, and the most frequent endocrine cause of neonatal death
      (b)   11β-hydroxylase deficiency – elevated serum 11-deoxycorticosterone and 11-deoxycortisol
      (c)   3β-hydroxysteroid dehydrogenase deficiency – elevated 17-hydroxypregnenolone and dehydroepiandrosterone
(2)   Male pseudohermaphroditism – the result of rare enzyme disorders
(3)   True hermaphrodite or gonadal dysgenesis – normal androgens, normal 17-OHP
      Laparotomy, gonadal biopsy, and/or gonadectomy is needed to confirm the diagnosis

TREATMENT

It is better to delay sex assignment, than to reverse it at a later date. Tell the parents that the genitals are unfinished, rather than abnormal

The sex assignment depends on whether the phallus can develop into a functional penis. The construction of female genitalia is technically easier

If reassignment of sex is necessary, it can usually be made safely up to 18 months of age

AMENORRHEA

DEFINITION (in absence of pregnancy)

(1)   No menses by age 14 in absence of secondary sexual characteristics, **or**

(2)   No menses by age 16 regardless of presence of secondary sexual characteristics, **or**

(3)   Three normal cycle intervals without menses or 6 months of amenorrhea in previously menstruating women

COMPARTMENTALIZATION OF EVALUATION

Compartment I: Outflow tract/endometrium
Compartment II: Ovary
Compartment III: Anterior pituitary
Compartment IV: CNS (hypothalamus)

EVALUATION

History & physical
R/o pregnancy
Therapeutic/laboratory investigation
TSH – r/o hypothyroidism
Prolactin – If greater than 100 mg/ml, MRI
Progestin challenge (progesterone in oil 200 mg IM or medroxyprogesterone acetate 10 mg p.o. q.d. x5 days)
     If + withdrawal bleed, diagnostic of anovulation
     If – withdrawal bleed, investigate Compartment I

COMPARTMENT I

Estrogen/progestin cycle (1.25 mg conjugated estrogen q.d. x21 days plus medroxyprogesterone acetate 10 mg q.d. for the last 5 days

Negative (–) withdrawal bleed   – defect in endometrium or outflow tract

Positive (+) withdrawal bleed   – investigate compartments II and IV

COMPARTMENTS II, III, and IV

FSH/LH assay – At least 2 wks after estrogen/progestin
     Low/normal – MRI   Hypothalamic amenorrhea
     High   Ovarian failure

AMENORRHEA

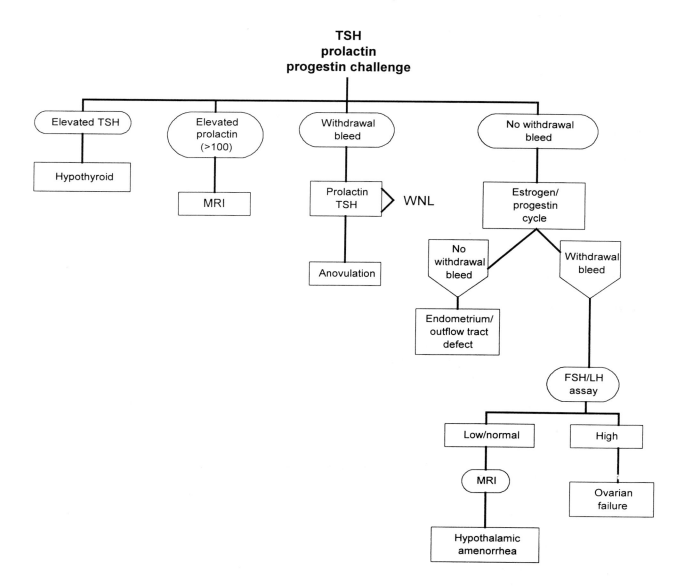

AMENORRHEA

NO MENSES BY AGE 14 YEARS, AND NO SECONDARY SEX CHARACTERISTICS
NO MENSES BY AGE 16 YEARS, WITH SECONDARY SEX CHARACTERISTICS

Patient type	Presumptions	Distinguishing tests
Breasts absent; uterus present	Lack of breasts indicates estrogen is not being produced by the gonads because of hypothalamic–pituitary failure, lack of ovarian follicles, or lack of two active X chromosomes Presence of uterus indicates Y chromosome is not present	FSH level identifies if estrogen lack is caused by ovarian failure (high FSH)* or hypothalamic–pituitary failure (low FSH) GnRH stimulation identifies whether the hypothalamus or pituitary has failed: • Hypothalamic failure (LH rises) • Pituitary failure (lack of LH response)
Breasts present; uterus absent	Presence of breasts indicates estrogen was or is being produced by the gonads Absence of uterus indicates either of the following: • Müllerian agenesis is present in an otherwise normal female (Mayer-Rokitansky) • The patient has a Y chromosome (androgen insensitivity)	Testosterone level suggests if the patient is: • 46XX with Müllerian agenesis (female levels) • 46XY with androgen insensitivity (male levels) Karyotyping confirms genetic sex is male with lack of androgen receptors. The gonads should be removed to prevent malignant transformation
Breasts absent; uterus absent	Lack of breasts indicates estrogen is not being produced by the gonads because of gonadal agenesis, agonadism, or rare gonadal enzyme deficiencies Absence of uterus indicates the patient has a Y chromosome with testes that produced MIF at one time Presence of female external genitalia indicates no testes were present to produce testosterone when the external genitalia formed	Karyotyping of 46XY, an elevated gonadotropin level and a testosterone level in the female range confirms gonadal agenesis of agonadism Gonadal biopsy is needed to diagnose rare enzyme deficiencies
Breasts present; uterus present	Presence of breasts indicates estrogen was or is being produced by the gonads Presence of uterus indicates Y chromosome is not present	These patients should be worked up with β-hCG, TSH level, prolactin level, progesterone challenge test

*High FSH: 99.00%, ovarian failure; 0.99%, 17-hydroxylase deficiency (46XX); 0.01%, oat cell CA of lung

AMNIOCENTESIS

DEFINITION

Amniocentesis is prenatal diagnostic testing of the amniotic fluid

GENETIC AMNIOCENTESIS

Gestation of 16–18 wks is the optimal time for genetic amniocentesis for the following indications:
(1)   Maternal age of 35 or older at EDC
(2)   Parental translocation carriers prior infant
(3)   Family history of neural tube defect
(4)   Paternal age of 55 years or older
(5)   Mother known to be carrier of X-linked disorder
(6)   History of habitual abortion
(7)   Risk for prenatally diagnosable biochemical/genetic disorder
(8)   Maternal serum fetoprotein abnormal

NON-GENETIC AMNIOCENTESIS

During the 2nd and 3rd half of pregnancy for the following indications:
(1)   Fetal lung maturity
(2)   Rh iso-immunization
(3)   Meconium
(4)   Postdatism
(5)   Amnionitis – for Gram stain and culture

PROCEDURE

(1)   Genetic counseling and informed patient consent must precede amniocentesis
(2)   The amniocentesis is to be performed by a physician
(3)   The amniocentesis is performed under aseptic technique. Select the site for transabdominal insertion of spinal needle (22 or 20 gauge) by ultrasonographic determination of placenta site, fetal position and the presence of a suitable pool of amniotic fluid. Avoid the placenta and fetus. All amniocentesis procedures are to be performed under sonographic guidance. The tap should be done, if possible, at midline to avoid major vessels
(4)   When an inadequate specimen is retrieved or the fluid is very bloody, a second needle insertion may be necessary. More than two needle insertions should be avoided. The first few drops of fluid should be discarded in order to minimize the risk of contamination by maternal cells in the needle pathway
(5)   In case of twins, one sac should be tapped, the fluid collected and 0.5 cc violet gentian should be inside the same sac. A second needle and another site should be used for the second tap. Clear fluid should be obtained
(6)   Patients are released after a brief period of observation and ultrasound documentation of fetal viability
(7)   Instructions should be given to patient about resting for the remainder of the day and notify in case of fever, contractions or bleeding

AMNIONITIS

DEFINITION

Amnionitis is a clinically defined infectious disease process involving the intrauterine contents during pregnancy. Synonymous terms include chorioamnionitis ("chorio"), intra-amniotic infection, and amniotic fluid infection.

For the most part, amnionitis is a bacterially mediated event, although other types of pathogens – such as mycoplasmas and viruses have been implicated as causative agents.

PATHOGENESIS

The most common route for infection involves the passage of micro-organisms from the lower genital tract in an ascending fashion. In a majority of cases, this follows either spontaneous or artificial rupture of the fetal membranes.

A less common route for transmission involves the hematogenous spread of a maternally derived organism via transplacental passage. The exact mechanism by which this occurs has yet to be clearly defined.

Organisms such as Group B streptococci and *Escherichia coli* are overly represented in amnionitis cases, in particular those associated with bacteremia. Organisms such as *Gardnerella vaginalis*, *Fusobacterium*, and *Bacteroides bivius* are not uncommonly seen in this disease process.

DIAGNOSIS

Criteria for the diagnosis of amnionitis include fever, maternal tachycardia, fetal tachycardia, uterine tenderness, foul-smelling amniotic fluid, and maternal leukocytosis. From a practical standpoint, fever is the primary clinical feature needed to establish the diagnosis of amnionitis.

The only laboratory studies that help support the diagnosis of amnionitis involve sampling of the amniotic fluid. Although culture is the gold standard for confirming the diagnosis, it is not particularly useful in the acute setting. A positive Gram stain (defined as the identification of any bacteria in an uncentrifuged amniotic fluid sample using high-power magnification) correlates relatively well with subsequent culture positivity.

THERAPY

When clinical amnionitis is diagnosed, basic goals of therapy are:
  (1)   To initiate the labor and delivery process regardless of the gestational age
  (2)   To attempt identification of the pathogens involved in the infectious disease process
  (3)   To initiate empiric antibiotic therapy
  (4)   To carefully monitor uterine and fetal heart rate activity

Given the mixed polymicrobial infectious disease process, broad spectrum parenteral antimicrobial therapy is indicated. This typically includes:
  (a)   Ampicillin, 1–2 g every 6 hrs
  (b)   Gentamicin given in loading and maintenance doses according to the patient's weight, and
  (c)   Clindamycin 900 mg every 8 hrs (or metronidazole)

In patients with mild to moderate infections use of any of the monotherapies seems appropriate (especially second- and third-generation cephalosporins and penicillins).

Unless delivery is imminent, it is recommended that antibiotic therapy be initiated during the intrapartum interval. Although this may hamper the neonate's evaluation with regard to sepsis, data clearly indicates an improvement in maternal and neonatal outcome when therapy is initiated early.

To reduce puerperal morbidity, the vaginal route is clearly preferable for the mother. For the fetus, vaginal delivery is preferred only if it is expeditious and atraumatic.

Patients with amnionitis usually have a prompt clinical response to delivery and antibiotics therapy. Assuming the patient has a rapid response to initial therapy, it would seem appropriate to discontinue antibiotics after the patient has been afebrile for 24 hrs, has return of bowel function, and does not demonstrate unusual uterine tenderness. If fever persists after delivery, the patient should be evaluated for other foci of infection or for associated non-infectious complications, such as septic pelvic thrombophlebitis.

DIAGNOSIS & MANAGEMENT OF AMNIONITIS

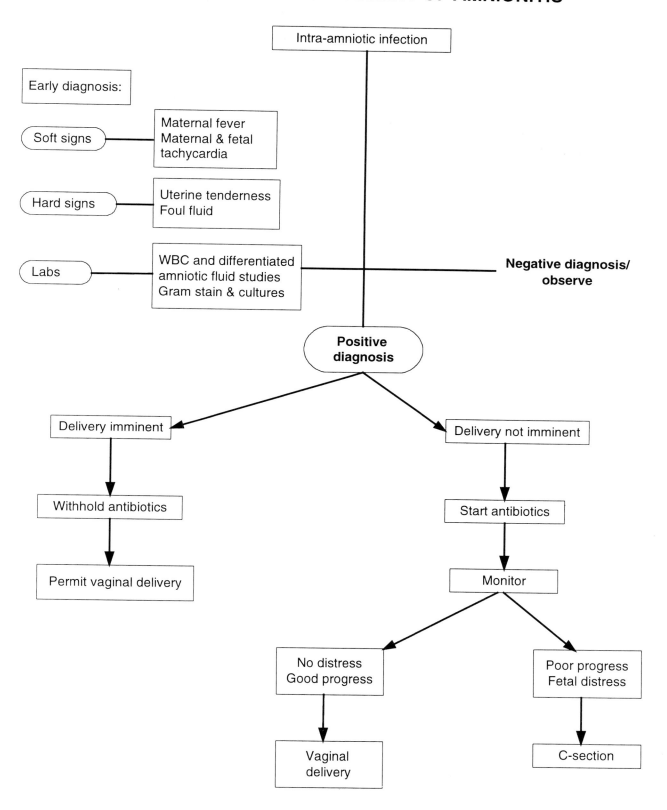

Intra-amniotic infection

Early diagnosis:

Soft signs —— Maternal fever
Maternal & fetal tachycardia

Hard signs —— Uterine tenderness
Foul fluid

Labs —— WBC and differentiated amniotic fluid studies
Gram stain & cultures

Negative diagnosis/ observe

Positive diagnosis

Delivery imminent

Delivery not imminent

Withhold antibiotics

Start antibiotics

Permit vaginal delivery

Monitor

No distress
Good progress

Poor progress
Fetal distress

Vaginal delivery

C-section

AMNIOTIC FLUID EMBOLISM

SUDDEN SIGNS

    (1)   Agitation
    (2)   Dyspnea
    (3)   Anxiety
    (4)   Respiratory arrest

During labor, delivery or postpartum

DIFFERENTIAL DIAGNOSIS

    (1)   Acute pulmonary edema
    (2)   Pulmonary emboli from the peripheral venous circulation
    (3)   Cardiac arrhythmias (MI)
    (4)   Uterine rupture or anesthesia complications can mimic

During resuscitative efforts – obtain blood from the pulmonary artery via central lines. Look for fetal squames (Attwood stain) and mucin (Giemsa stain). This will confirm the diagnosis in patients that survive

MANAGEMENT

    (1)   Endotracheal intubation
    (2)   ABGs (monitor for blood gases to maintain O_2 flow rates)
    (3)   CPR p.r.n.
    (4)   Digoxin or dopamine (in 2nd phase of disorder for left ventricular failure)
    (5)   Swan–Ganz (triple-lumen pulmonary artery) catheter (Obtain special stains during placement)
    (6)   ICU (if patient survives – meticulous attention to cardiac and renal function and fluid balance)
    (7)   Pay attention to blood loss (PTT, plts, FDP, fibrinogen)
    (8)   FFP and/or plts for D/C

AMNIOTIC FLUID EMBOLISM

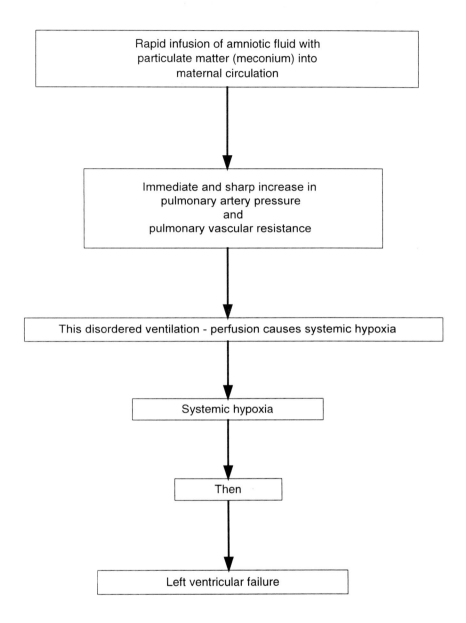

Rapid infusion of amniotic fluid with
particulate matter (meconium) into
maternal circulation

Immediate and sharp increase in
pulmonary artery pressure
and
pulmonary vascular resistance

This disordered ventilation - perfusion causes systemic hypoxia

Systemic hypoxia

Then

Left ventricular failure

*Thromboplastin-rich amniotic fluid triggers the intrinsic
clotting system with rapid defibrination and hemorrhage (DIC)
which aggravates an already complex cardiovascular picture*

BREAKTHROUGH BLEEEDING

BREAKTHROUGH BLEEDING – COMPLICATIONS FOR WOMEN ON OCPs

(a)   More likely to occur in smokers than non-smokers
(b)   Taking OCPs at same time each day minimizes BTB
(c)   Pelvic infections may also cause BTB. Evaluate p.r.n.

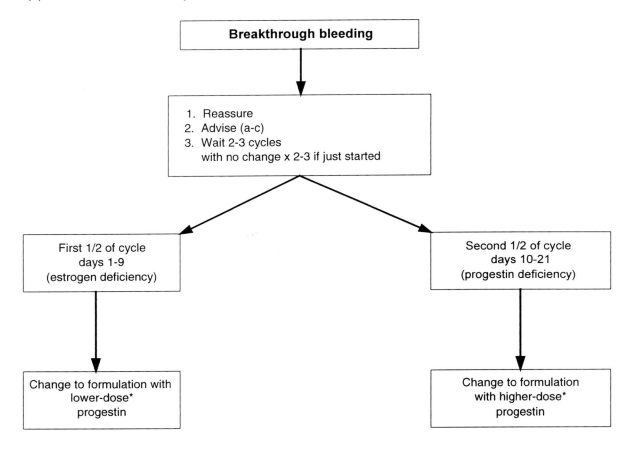

* See contraceptive dosages

BREAST

TYPES OF NIPPLE DISCHARGE

Color	Other names	Most common cause	Frequency	% Caused by cancer
Milky	Galactorrhea	Physiologic Breast-feeding Pregnancy Postpartum Prolactin excess Pituitary adenomas		Unknown
Multicolored	Sticky, green yellow, serous	Ductal ectasia		Rare
Purulent	Infected	Bacterial infection		Rare
Clear	Watery	Ductal carcinoma	2.2%	33.3–45%
Yellow	Serous	Fibrocystic disease	41.1%	5.9%
Pink	Serosanguinous	Fibrocystic disease Ductal papillomas	31.8%	12.9%
Bloody	Sanguinous	Fibrocystic disease Ductal papillomas	24.9%	27%

BREAST MASS
Diagnosis & treatment

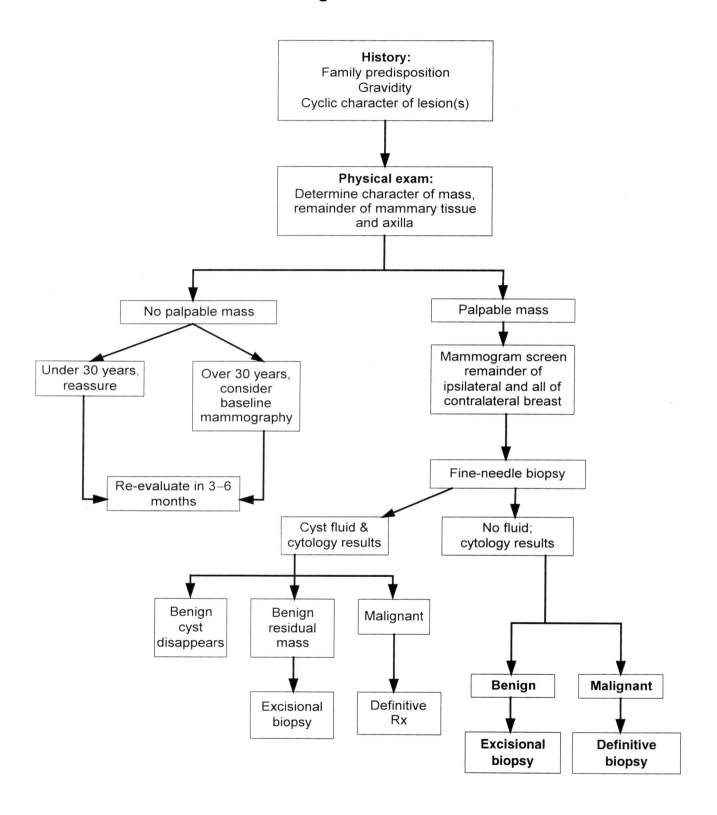

History:
Family predisposition
Gravidity
Cyclic character of lesion(s)

Physical exam:
Determine character of mass,
remainder of mammary tissue
and axilla

No palpable mass

Palpable mass

Under 30 years,
reassure

Over 30 years,
consider
baseline
mammography

Mammogram screen
remainder of
ipsilateral and all of
contralateral breast

Re-evaluate in 3–6
months

Fine-needle biopsy

Cyst fluid &
cytology results

No fluid;
cytology results

Benign
cyst
disappears

Benign
residual
mass

Malignant

Excisional
biopsy

Definitive
Rx

Benign

Malignant

**Excisional
biopsy**

**Definitive
biopsy**

NIPPLE DISCHARGE

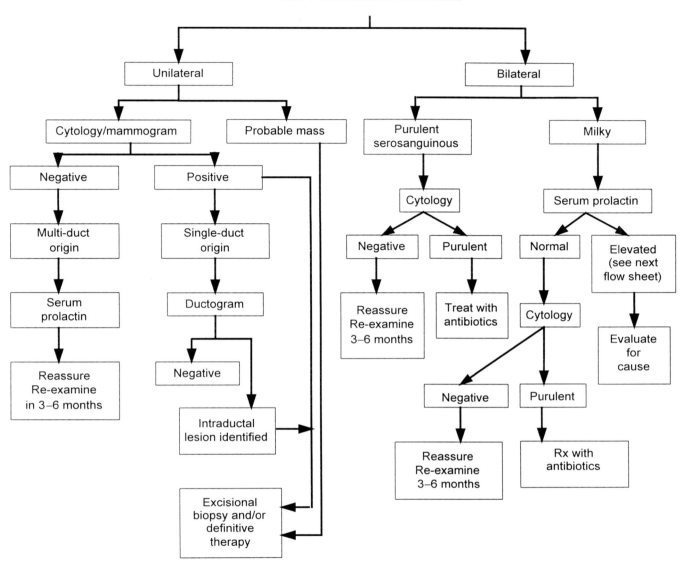

NIPPLE DISCHARGE
*Hyperprolactinemia

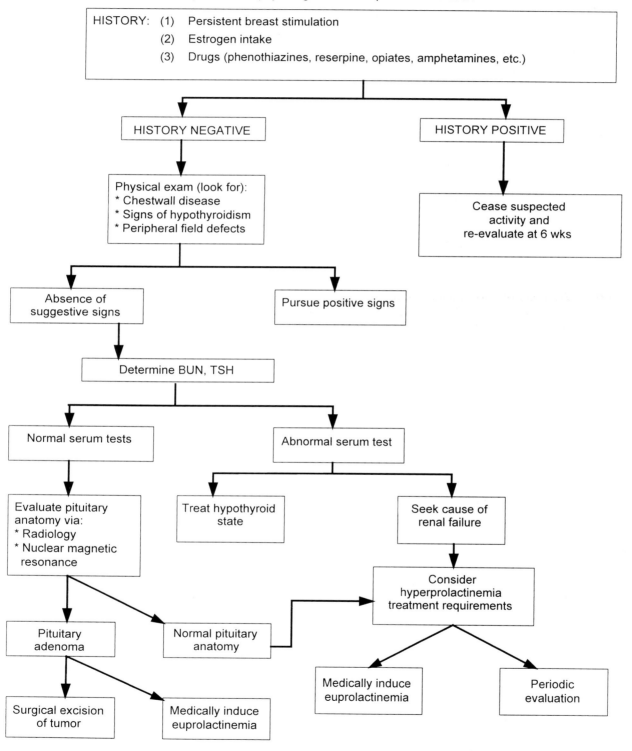

Repeat serum assay to rule out physiologic causes of prolactin secretion

HISTORY: (1) Persistent breast stimulation
(2) Estrogen intake
(3) Drugs (phenothiazines, reserpine, opiates, amphetamines, etc.)

HISTORY NEGATIVE

HISTORY POSITIVE

Physical exam (look for):
* Chestwall disease
* Signs of hypothyroidism
* Peripheral field defects

Cease suspected activity and re-evaluate at 6 wks

Absence of suggestive signs

Pursue positive signs

Determine BUN, TSH

Normal serum tests

Abnormal serum test

Evaluate pituitary anatomy via:
* Radiology
* Nuclear magnetic resonance

Treat hypothyroid state

Seek cause of renal failure

Pituitary adenoma

Normal pituitary anatomy

Consider hyperprolactinemia treatment requirements

Surgical excision of tumor

Medically induce euprolactinemia

Medically induce euprolactinemia

Periodic evaluation

BREAST

PUERPERAL MASTITIS (3 categories)

(1) *Milk stasis* – incomplete breast emptying causing engorgement and pain
(2) *Non-infectious inflammation* – arises when milk stasis is persistent and severe leading to edema, erythema, pain and tenderness
(3) *Acute mastitis* – final step in progression of disease characterized by: edema, erythema, pain, myalgias, chills, fever, tenderness

Predisposing factors

(1) Failure to empty breast adequately, most common
(2) Fissuring of nipples and bacterial inoculum from infant's mouth/mother's skin
(3) Incorrect preparation/care of nipples
(4) Improper positioning of infant for nursing
(5) Lowered maternal immune defenses

Diagnosis (acute puerperal mastitis)

(1) Symptoms: malaise, myalgias, fever, chills, pain
(2) Signs: edema, erythema, temp >37.8 °C (100 °F), breast tenderness
(3) Milk cultures (discard first 3 cc)
   (a) Milk stasis: $<10^6$ leukocytes/cc; $<10^3$ bacteria/cc
   (b) Non-infectious inflammation: $>10^6$ leukocytes/cc, $<10^3$ bacteria/cc
   (c) Infectious mastitis: $>10^6$ leukocytes/cc, $>10^3$ bacteria/cc

Treatment

(1) Adequate milk emptying (continued nursing, infection extraductal)
(2) Moist heat
(3) Adequate hydration
(4) NSAIDs (ibuprofen, Naprosyn, etc.)
(5) Empiric antibiotics:
   (a) Dicloxacillin 500 mg p.o. q. 6 hrs
   (b) Ampicillin 500 mg p.o. q. 6 hrs
   (c) Erythromycin 500 mg p.o. q. 6 hrs
   (d) Cephalexin 500 mg p.o. q. 6 hrs

Sequelae

(1) Persistent infection/breast abscess
(2) Increased risk if nursing discontinued
(3) Once diagnosed:
   (a) Cease nursing on infected side
   (b) Initiate IV antibiotics
      – ancef 1 g IV q. 6–8 hrs, or
      – ampicillin 1 g IV q. 6 hrs
        AND
      – clindamycin 900 mg IV q. 8 hrs, or
      – metronidazole 500 mg IV q. 6 hrs
        OR
      – unasyn 1.5–3.0 g IV q. 6 hrs
(4) Absence of favorable response within 48–72 hrs requires surgical I&D

NONPUERPERAL MASTITIS

Characterized as partial blockage of ducts by keratotic debris and squamous metaplasia

Predisposing factors

(1)   Manipulation of breast (mammogram)
(2)   Oral stimulation
(3)   Adjacent cutaneous infection

Diagnosis

(1)   *Acute –* pain, fever, edema, erythema, firm subareolar mass
(2)   *Subacute –* similar presentation with tender, fluctuant mass
(3)   *Chronic –* follows multiple, recurrent infections (sinus tracts, suppuration, fluctuant mass, pain and edema)

Treatment

(1)   *Acute –* penicillinase-resistant penicillin plus metronidazole, or broad-spectrum antibiotic (fluoroquinolone)
(2)   *Subacute –* surgical I&D, broad spectrum antibiotics

CARDIAC DEFECTS

MANAGEMENT OF CARDIAC VALVE DEFECTS IN GRAVIDAS

Lesion	Pathophysiology	Maternal complications	Key to therapy	Endocarditis prophylaxis*
Mitral stenosis	Limited left ventricular filling	Arrhythmia, pulmonary congestion	Optimize preload; avoid hypotension and tachycardia	Recommended
Mitral insufficiency	Atrial regurgitation	Limited cardiac output, arrhythmia, pulmonary congestion	Avoid hypotension and tachycardia	Optional
Aortic stenosis	Obstructed left ventricular outflow	Fixed cardiac output, compromised blood supply to coronary and cerebral arteries	Maintain cardiac output; reduce afterload; avoid hypotension and tachycardia	Recommended
Aortic insufficiency	Regurgitant cardiac output	Limited cardiac output, congestive heart failure	Avoid volume overload; reduce afterload	Recommended

MANAGEMENT OF STRUCTURAL CARDIAC DEFECTS IN GRAVIDAS

Lesion	Pathophysiology	Maternal complications	Key to therapy	Endocarditis prophylaxis*
Atrial septal defect	Bidirectional atrial flow	Arrhythmia	Avoid volume overload	Recommended
Ventricular septal defect	Left-to-right shunt	Right ventricular overload	Avoid volume overload	No
Patent ductus arteriosus	Left-to-right shunt	Increased pulmonary flow	Avoid volume overload	Recommended
Eisenmenger syndrome	Pulmonary hypertension with bidirectional shunting	Congestive heart failure, hypoxia, sudden death	Recommended termination of pregnancy; supply continuous oxygen; avoid hypotension	Recommended
Tetralogy of Fallot	Ventricular septal defect, overriding aorta, pulmonary stenosis, and right-to-left shunt	Congestive heart failure, hypoxia	Maintain preload delivery with limited afterload reduction; provide oxygen	Recommended
Coarctation of the aorta	Obstructed cardiac output	Limited cardiac output, congestive heart failure, aortic dissection or rupture	Reduce afterload; avoid volume overload	Recommended

MANAGEMENT OF DEVELOPMENTAL CARDIAC VALVE DEFECTS IN GRAVIDAS

Lesion	Pathophysiology	Maternal complications	Key to therapy	Endocarditis prophylaxis*
Idiopathic hyper-trophic subaortic	Obstructed outflow from left ventricle	Fixed cardiac output, congestive heart failure	Obstruction improves with volume expansion; avoid hypotension and tachycardia	Recommended
Marfan's syndrome	Aortic regurgitation with aneurysm formation at the aortic root	Aortic dissection or rupture, marginal cardiac output, congestive heart failure secondary to regurgitation	Maintain cardiac output; avoid volume overload; prescribe beta-blockers	Recommended

*Endocarditis prophylaxis: ampicillin 2 g IV, then 1 g q. 4–6 hrs while in labor; gentamycin 1.5 mg/kg IV then repeated 8 hrs later

CARDIAC DEFECTS

LETHAL DYSRHYTHMIA PROTOCOLS

Ventricular fibrillation

Defibrillate at 200–300 J. Repeat if ineffective

Intubate and ventilate with oxygen. Give epinephrine, 0.5–1.0 mg IV. Repeat every 5 min. Give sodium bicarbonate, 1 mEq/kg (75–100 mg). Repeat with half the dose every 10 min as needed

Defibrillate at 360 J; repeat

Give bretylium tosylate (Bretylol), 5 mg/kg IV (350–500 mg)

Defibrillate at 360 J; repeat

Give bretylium, 10 mg/kg IV (750–1000 mg)

Defibrillate at 360 J; repeat

After the maximum dose of bretylium, or as an alternative, one may give lidocaine hydrochloride (Xylocaine) or procainamide hydrochloride (Pronestyl) as an adjunct to defibrillation

Give 1 mg/kg of lidocaine as an initial bolus, and follow after 10 min by 0.5 mg/kg. This may be repeated until a total dose of 225 mg is reached, and followed by maintenance infusion at 2–4 mg/min

Give 100 mg of procainamide over 5 min, repeated every 5 min. Stop bolus dosage on noting hypotension, suppression of dysrhythmia, a 50% increase in width of the QRS complex, or on reaching a total dose of 1 g. Maintenance is 1–4 mg/min

Asystole

Intubate and ventilate with oxygen. Give epinephrine, 0.5–1.0 mg IV. Repeat every 5 min. Give sodium bicarbonate, 1 mEq/kg (75–100 mg). Repeat with half the dose every 10 min as needed

Give atropine 1.0 mg IV

Give calcium chloride 10% solution, 5 ml IV. Repeat every 10 min

Give isoproterenol (Isuprel) infusion, 2–20 mg/min

Arrange for pacemaker placement

Electromechanical dissociation

Intubate and ventilate with oxygen. Give epinephrine 0.5–1.0 mg IV. Repeat every 5 min. Give sodium bicarbonate, 1 mEq/kg (75–100 mEq). Repeat half the dose every 10 min as needed

Give calcium chloride, 10% solution IV 5 ml. Repeat every 10 min

Give isoproterenol infusion, 2–20 mg/min

Consider hypovolemia, tension pneumothorax, and cardiac tamponade as possible causes, and treat appropriately

CARPAL TUNNEL SYNDROME

DIAGNOSIS

Paresthesias, pain, numbness or loss of manual dexterity. Nocturnal exacerbation, weakness of grasp, decreased dexterity, night pain in wrist and hand

Classic CTS symptoms: radial 3 digits with localized numbness and tingling

Tinel's test

Tap over transverse carpal ligament – produces tingling in fingers
+Tinel's sign

Phalen's (wrist flexion) test

Elbows are placed on flat surface with forearms held in vertical position; then wrists are acutely flexed. Positive (+) if pain, numbness, or tingling is produced or exacerbated within 60 seconds (+ in 60% of patients)

EMG if ?

Cervical disc herniation, MS, neuropathies, polyneuritis

X-rays if history of trauma or older patient with osteoarthritis

Rx

Non-pregnant or
Pregnancy (swelling, hormonal changes)
Splinting, vitamin B_6 100 mg daily; local steroid injection (1 ml or 40 mg) of Depo-Medrol with 1 ml of 1% lidocaine without epinephrine
Surgery only if necessary

ASSOCIATED CONDITIONS AND CAUSES

Trauma-related structural changes	Systemic diseases	Hormonal changes	Tumors/ neoplasms	Anomalous anatomic structures	Mechanical overuse	Infections
Distal radius fracture	Rheumatoid conditions: arthritis, gout, cervical atrophy, intercarpal arteritis, tenosynovitis, bursitis, fibromyositis	Pregnancy	Lipoma	Aberrant muscles (e.g. lumbrical, palmaris longus, palmaris profundus)	Vibrating machinery	Tuberculosis (and other mycobacterial infections)
Lunate/ perilunate dislocations	Diabetes mellitus	Acromegaly	Ganglion	Median artery thrombosis	Prolonged hammering	Pyogenic infections
Post-traumatic arthritis/ osteophytes	Thyroid imbalance (especially hypothyroid)	Menopause	Multiple myeloma	Enlarged persistent median artery	Prolonged typing	Leprosy
Edema	Amyloidosis	Oral contraceptive use	Vascular tumors	Hypertrophy of palmaris longus muscle		
Hemorrhage/ hematoma	Hemophilia	Systemic steroid use		Arteriovenous fistulas (hemodialysis)		
Burns	Alcoholism/ cirrhosis					
Colles' fracture	Raynaud's phenomenon, Paget's disease, obesity, syphilis, acromegaly, Cushing's disease, sarcoidosis, systemic lupus erythematosus, polymyositis, scleroderma, pernicious anemia, adiposita dolorosa, purpura simplex					

CERVICAL INCOMPETENCE

DIAGNOSIS

Characterized by painless dilatation of the cervix in the second (or early third) trimester
May be associated with bulging membranes and eventually, rupture of membranes followed by expulsion of a premature fetus

ETIOLOGY

Previous cervical trauma (D&C, conization, cauterization, amputation, obstetrical injury)
DES exposure/uterine anomalies

PREVENTION

Use of tapered dilators
Use of laminaria (especially in nulliparous patients)
Experienced operator

PRE-OPERATIVE EVALUATION

Delayed until 14 wks EGA (early SABs completed)
Seldom performed after 20 wks (not after 26 wks)
Ultrasound (r/o major anomalies, confirm viability)
Screen for: GC, *Chlamydia* & Group B Strep
     Treat for positive cultures prior to procedure
Confirm negative cervical cytology
Sexual abstinence at least one week before and one week after procedure

TREATMENT

Cerclage (McDonald, Shirodkar, abdominal)
   McDonald – procedure of choice
      – Purse-string technique using 5 mm Merselene band
      – 4–5 "bites" at level of internal os
      – Knot placed anteriorly (facilitates removal)
   Shirodkar – more difficult
      – Used with previous McDonald failures
      – Submucosal placement (bladder mobilized cephalad)
      – More closely approaches level of internal os
   Special considerations
      – Elevation of bulging membranes
         (1) Overfill bladder with 1000 cc saline
         (2) Trendelenberg (with or without Foley displacement)
      – Short or amputated cervix – abdominal cerclage

COMPLICATIONS

Much less common when performed before 18 wks EGA
  (1)   Rupture of membranes – remove cerclage/induce labor
  (2)   Chorioamnionitis – amniocentesis to confirm – remove/induce
  (3)   Preterm labor – use of tocolysis or antibiotics pre-op until 24 hrs
        post-op may reduce risk*

Failure to remove cerclage may result in uterine/cervical rupture
Shirodkar/abdominal cerclage difficult or impossible to remove often requiring C-section

  *According to operator's preference

CHOLESTEROL MANAGEMENT

NATIONAL CHOLESTEROL EDUCATION PROGRAM – GUIDELINES AND GOALS FOR YOUR PATIENTS AT RISK

When diet and exercise are not enough to lower cholesterol, the NCEP recommends lowering LDL-cholesterol following the guidelines below. Using these levels and risk factors as guidelines, medications such as atorvastatin (Lipitor), fluvastatin, pravastatin, simvastatin, or lovestatin may be started

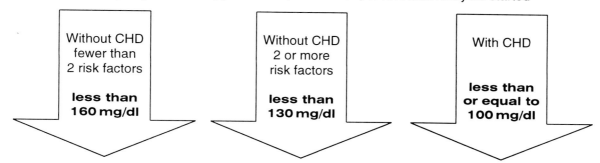

Without CHD
fewer than
2 risk factors

**less than
160 mg/dl**

Without CHD
2 or more
risk factors

**less than
130 mg/dl**

With CHD

**less than
or equal to
100 mg/dl**

NCEP recommends lowering LDL-C further than these goals if possible

IDENTIFYING PATIENTS WITH CHD RISK FACTORS

Family history of early CHD

Any parent or sibling with CHD (younger than 55 years if male and younger than 65 years if female)

Age

Male ≥45 years; female ≥55 years or premature menopause without estrogen replacement therapy
– Men in their forties are four times more likely to die from CHD than women of the same age. After menopause, the incidence of CHD increases progressively in women until ultimately as many women as men die of CHD

Hypertension

Blood pressure ≥40/90 mmHg or on antihypertensive medication
– Because it is difficult to determine how long blood pressure has been controlled vs uncontrolled, even patients undergoing treatment are considered to be at risk

Current smoker

Smoking cessation is one of the most effective ways to reduce the risk of CHD and other atherosclerotic diseases

Diabetes mellitus

In men, diabetes triples the risk of CHD; in women, the increase in risk may be even greater

Low HDL-cholesterol (<3.5 mg/dl)

Evidence shows that for every 1-mg/dl decrease in HDL-C, the risk of CHD is increased by 2–3%. In the Framingham study, a 10-mg/dl decrease in HDL-C correlated to a 50% increase in coronary risk among women

If HDL-C is ≥60 mg/dl, subtract one risk factor

Indicated as an adjunct to diet to reduce elevated total cholesterol (TC), LDL-C, apoB, and TG levels in patients with primary hypercholesterolemia (heterozygous familial and nonfamilial) and mixed dyslipidemia

CHOLESTEROL MANAGEMENT

Primary prevention in adults without evidence of CHD:

initial classification based on total cholesterol and HDL-cholesterol

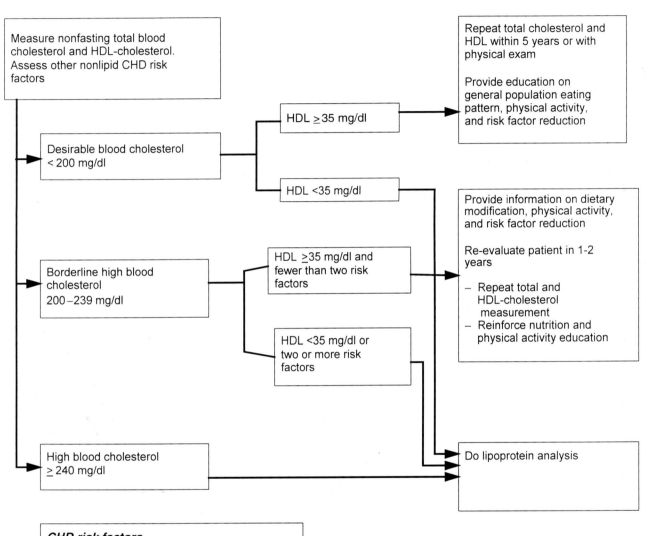

Measure nonfasting total blood cholesterol and HDL-cholesterol. Assess other nonlipid CHD risk factors

Desirable blood cholesterol < 200 mg/dl

HDL ≥ 35 mg/dl

HDL < 35 mg/dl

Borderline high blood cholesterol 200 – 239 mg/dl

HDL ≥ 35 mg/dl and fewer than two risk factors

HDL < 35 mg/dl or two or more risk factors

High blood cholesterol ≥ 240 mg/dl

Repeat total cholesterol and HDL within 5 years or with physical exam

Provide education on general population eating pattern, physical activity, and risk factor reduction

Provide information on dietary modification, physical activity, and risk factor reduction

Re-evaluate patient in 1-2 years

- Repeat total and HDL-cholesterol measurement
- Reinforce nutrition and physical activity education

Do lipoprotein analysis

CHD risk factors

Positive
Age: Male ≥ 45 years
          Female ≥ 55 years or premature menopause without estrogen replacement therapy
Family history of premature CHD
Smoking
Hypertension
HDL-cholesterol <35 mg/dl
Diabetes

Negative
HDL-cholesterol ≥ 60 mg/dl

CHOLESTEROL MANAGEMENT

Primary prevention in adults without evidence of CHD:
subsequent classification based on LDL-cholesterol

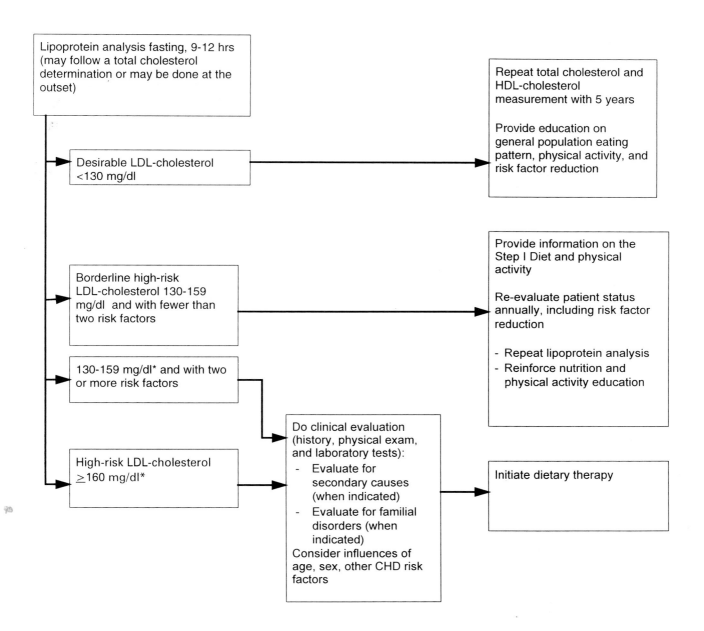

*On the basis of the average of two determinations. If the first two LDL-cholesterol tests differ by more than 30 mg/dl, a third test should be obtained within 1-8 weeks and the average value of three tests used

CHOLESTEROL MANAGEMENT

Secondary prevention in adults with evidence of CHD: classification based on LDL-cholesterol

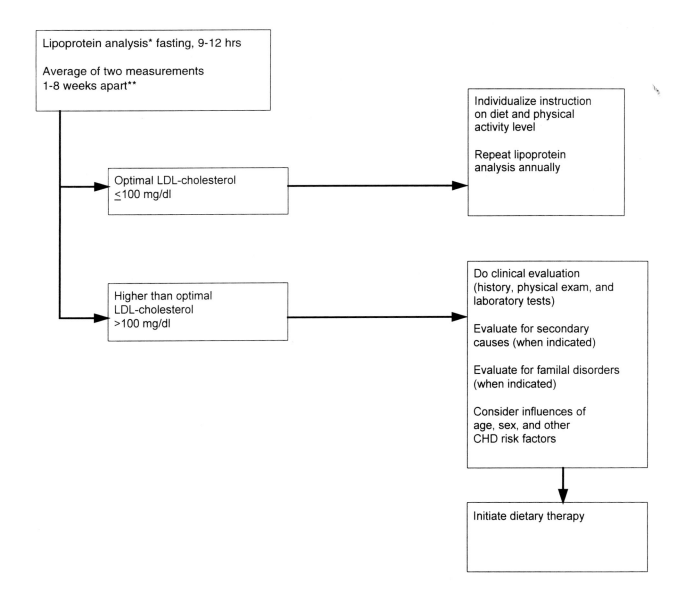

Lipoprotein analysis* fasting, 9-12 hrs

Average of two measurements 1-8 weeks apart**

Optimal LDL-cholesterol ≤100 mg/dl

Individualize instruction on diet and physical activity level

Repeat lipoprotein analysis annually

Higher than optimal LDL-cholesterol >100 mg/dl

Do clinical evaluation (history, physical exam, and laboratory tests)

Evaluate for secondary causes (when indicated)

Evaluate for familal disorders (when indicated)

Consider influences of age, sex, and other CHD risk factors

Initiate dietary therapy

* Lipoprotein analysis should be performed when the patient is not in the recovery phase from an acute coronary or other medical event that would lower their usual LDL-cholesterol level

** If the first two LDL-cholesterol tests differ by more than 30 mg/dl, a third test should be obtained within 1-8 wks and the average value of the three tests used

CONTRACEPTION

POSTCOITAL REGIMENS

Norgestrel and ethinyl estradiol: 2 tablets immediately, then 2 more tablets 12 hrs later

Levonorgestrel and ethinyl estradiol; 4 yellow tablets immediately, then 4 more yellow tablets 12 hrs later

Levonorgestrel and ethinyl estradiol (triphasic regimen): 4 yellow tablets immediately, then 4 more yellow tablets 12 hrs later

Ethinyl estradiol: 2.5 mg b.i.d. or 5 mg daily for 4 days

Conjugated estrogens: 30 mg daily for 5 days, 10 mg for 5 days, or 25 mg IV immediately and 25 mg 24 hrs later

Estrone: 5 mg b.i.d. for 5 days

Danazol: 400–600 mg immediately, then repeated 12 hrs later

Copper IUD: insert within 5–7 days of exposure (except in cases of rape or STD infection)

Preven is now available to prescribe specifically for postcoital contraception in place of any of the above regimens

CONTRACEPTION

CONCERNS PRIOR TO STARTING ORAL CONTRACEPTIVES

Suggested screening examination

Blood pressure measurement
Breast, abdominal, and pelvic examination
Pap test
Complete blood count
Urinalysis
In case of family history of vascular disease: lipid panel
In case of family history of diabetes: 2-hr postprandial blood glucose test; if elevated, perform glucose tolerance test
In case of patient history of liver disease: liver panel

Contraindications and precautions to the use of oral contraceptives

Contraindications

Oral contraceptives should not be used by women who currently have the following conditions:

Thrombophlebitis or thromboembolic disorders
A history of deep vein thrombophlebitis or thromboembolic disorders
Cerebral vascular or coronary artery disease
Known or suspected carcinoma of the breast
Carcinoma of the endometrium or other known or suspected estrogen-dependent neoplasia
Undiagnosed abnormal genital bleeding
Cholestatic jaundice of pregnancy or jaundice with prior OC use
Hepatic adenomas or carcinomas
Known or suspected pregnancy

Precautions

Women with the following conditions who take oral contraceptives should be monitored with particular care:

Breast nodules or a strong family history of breast cancer
Hyperlipidemia
Impaired liver function
Conditions that may be aggravated by fluid retention
History of depression
Visual changes or changes in lens tolerance in a woman with contact lenses (should be assessed by an ophthalmologist)

MISSED PILLS

Preventing pregnancy in women who miss one or more oral contraceptive pill(s)

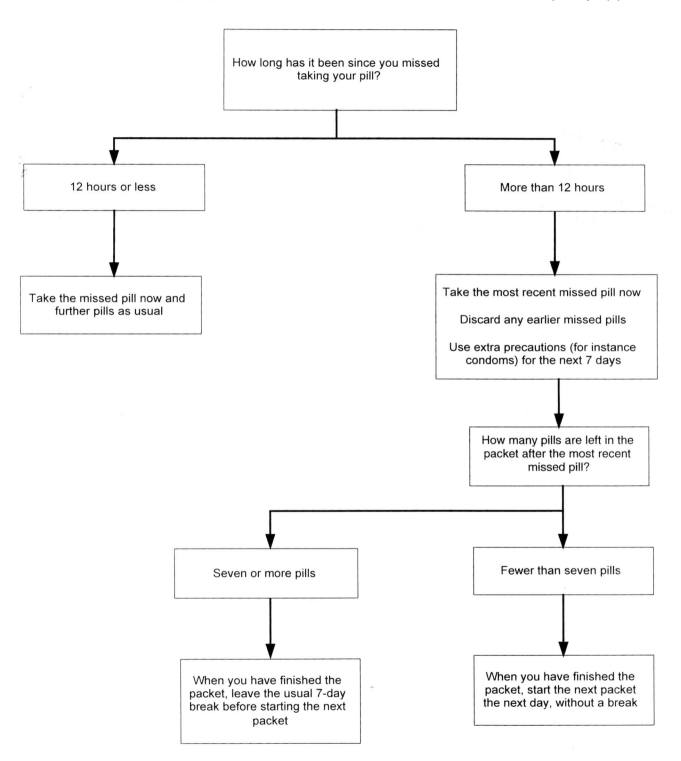

CONTRACEPTION

ORAL CONTRACEPTIVE TYPES AND DOSAGES

Low-dose monophasics

Alesse (Wyeth-Ayerst) 21 or 28 day
    0.1 mg levonorgestrel
    0.02 mg ethinyl estradiol
Brevicon (Searle) 21 or 28 day
    0.5 mg norethindrone
    0.035 mg ethinyl estradiol
Demulen 1/35 (Searle) 21 or 28 day
    1 mg ethynodiol diacetate
    35 µg ethinyl estradiol
Desogen (Organon) 28 day
    0.15 mg desogestrel
    0.03 mg ethinyl estradiol
Levlen (Berlex) 21 or 28 day
    0.15 mg levonorgestrel
    0.03 mg ethinyl estradiol
Loestrin 1/20 (Parke-Davis) 21 day
    1 mg norethindrone acetate
    20 µg ethinyl estradiol
Loestrin 1.5/30 (Parke-Davis) 21 day
    1.5 mg norethindrone acetate
    30 µg ethinyl estradiol
Loestrin Fe 1/20 (Parke-Davis) 28 day
    1 mg norethindrone acetate
    20 µg ethinyl estradiol
    7 pills 75 mg ferrous fumarate
Loestrin Fe 1.5/30 (Parke-Davis) 28 day
    1.5 mg norethindrone acetate
    30 µg ethinyl estradiol
    7 pills 75 mg ferrous fumarate
Lo-Ovral (Wyeth-Ayerst) 21 or 28 day
    0.3 mg norgestrel
    0.03 mg ethinyl estradiol
Mircette (Organon) 28 day
    20 µg ethinyl estradiol
    150 µg desogestrel (days 1–21)
    Placebo (days 22–23)
    10 µg ethinyl estradiol (days 24–28)
Modicon (Ortho) 21 or 28 day
    0.5 mg norethindrone
    0.035 mg ethinyl estradiol
Nelova 1/35E (Warner-Chilcott)
    1 mg norethindrone
    35 µg ethinyl estradiol
Nelova 0.5/35E (Warner-Chilcott)
    0.5 mg norethindrone
    35 µg ethinyl estradiol
Nordette (Wyeth-Ayerst) 21 or 28 day
    0.15 mg levonorgestrel
    0.03 mg ethinyl estradiol
Norethin 1/35E (Roberts) 28 day
    1 mg norethindrone
    35 µg ethinyl estradiol

Norinyl 1+35 (Searle) 21 or 28 day
    1 mg norethindrone
    0.035 mg ethinyl estradiol
Ortho-Cept (Ortho) 21 or 28 day
    0.15 mg desogestrel
    0.03 mg ethinyl estradiol
Ortho-Cyclen (Ortho) 21 or 28 day
    0.250 mg norgestimate
    0.035 mg ethinyl estradiol
Ortho-Novum 1/35 (Ortho) 21 or 28 day
    1 mg norethindrone
    0.035 mg ethinyl estradiol
Ovcon 35 (Bristol-Myers Squibb) 21 or 28 day
    0.4 mg norethindrone
    0.035 mg ethinyl estradiol

Triphasics

Ortho-Novum 7/7/7 (Ortho) 21 or 28 day
    7 days: 0.5 mg norethindrone
            0.035 mg ethinyl estradiol
    7 days: 0.75 mg norethindrone
            0.035 mg ethinyl estradiol
    7 days: 1 mg norethindrone
            0.035 mg ethinyl estradiol
Tri-Levlen (Berlex) 21 or 28 day
    6 days: 0.050 mg levonorgestrel
            0.030 mg ethinyl estradiol
    5 days: 0.075 mg levonorgestrel
            0.040 mg ethinyl estradiol
    10 days: 0.125 mg levonorgestrel
            0.030 mg ethinyl estradiol
Tri-Cyclen (Ortho) 21 or 28 day
    7 days: 0.180 mg norgestimate
            0.35 mg ethinyl estradiol
    7 days: 0.215 mg norgestimate
            0.035 mg ethinyl estradiol
    7 days: 0.250 mg norgestimate
            0.035 mg ethinyl estradiol
Tri-Norinyl (Searle) 21 or 28 day
    7 days: 0.5 mg norethindrone
            0.035 mg ethinyl estradiol
    9 days: 1 mg norethindrone
            0.035 mg ethinyl estradiol
    5 days: 0.5 mg norethindrone
            0.035 mg ethinyl estradiol
Triphasil (Wyeth-Ayerst) 21 or 28 day
    6 days: 0.050 mg levonorgestrel
            0.030 mg ethinyl estradiol
    5 days: 0.075 mg levonorgestrel
            0.040 mg ethinyl estradiol
    10 days: 0.125 mg levonorgestrel
            0.030 mg ethinyl estradiol

Biphasics

Jenest (Organon) 28 day
 7 days: 0.5 mg norethindrone
     0.035 mg ethinyl estradiol
 14 days: 1 mg norethindrone
     0.035 mg ethinyl estradiol
Ortho-Novum 10/11 (Ortho) 21 or 28 day
 10 days: 0.5 mg norethindrone
     0.035 mg ethinyl estradiol
 11 days: 1 mg norethindrone
     0.035 mg ethinyl estradiol

Graduated estrophasics

Estrostep 21 (Parke-Davis) 21 day
 5 days: 1 mg norethindrone acetate
     0.02 mg ethinyl estradiol
 7 days: 1 mg norethindrone acetate
     0.03 mg ethinyl estradiol
 9 days: 1 mg norethindrone acetate
     0.035 mg ethinyl estradiol
Estrostep FE (Parke-Davis) 28 day
 5 days: 1 mg norethindrone acetate
     0.02 mg ethinyl estradiol
 7 days: 1 mg norethindrone acetate
     0.03 mg ethinyl estradiol
 9 days: 1 mg norethindrone acetate
     0.035 mg ethinyl estradiol
 7 days: 75 mg ferrous fumarate

Progestin-only

Micronor (Ortho) 28 day
 0.35 mg norethindrone
Nor-QD (Searle) 42 day
 0.35 mg norethindrone
Ovrette (Wyeth-Ayerst) 28 day
 0.075 mg norgestrel

Adapted from Caufield KA. Controlling fertility. In Youngkin EQ, Davis MSD, eds. *Women's Health: A Primary Care Clinical Guide*. Norwalk, Connecticut: Appleton and Lange, 1994:112–14; and *Physician's Desk Reference*, 51st edn. Montvale, NJ: Medical Economics Books, 1997

CORD PROLAPSE

INCIDENCE

1/200

PERINATAL MORTALITY

2–8% (one source states over 20%)

PREDISPOSING FACTORS

(1) Most frequent causes
    (a) Abnormal presentation
    (b) Fetal hypotension (with abruptio)
    (c) Multiparity
    (d) Multiple gestation
    (e) Prematurity

(2) Less common factors
    (a) Contracted pelvis
    (b) Extended cord length
    (c) Obstetric manipulations
    (d) Polyhydramnios
    (e) Premature rupture of membranes
    (f) Rupture of membranes before engagement (spont. or art.)

DIAGNOSIS

(1) Palpable cord on vaginal exam

(2) Observed cord protruding onto vulva

(3) FHR pattern suggesting cord compression
    (a) Prolonged, severe, variable decelerations
    (b) Bradycardia
    (c) Ultrasound (may dx high-risk cases prior to distress)

MANAGEMENT

(1) Place mother in Trendelenburg or knee-chest position

(2) Elevate presenting fetal part

(3) Administer oxygen to mother

(4) Swiftly order preparations for C-section

(5) If preparations are prolonged:
    (a) Distend bladder (500–700 ml NS thru cath)
    (b) Administer a tocolytic agent (terbutaline) IV
    These steps will serve to elevate presenting part and decrease or stop uterine contractions both allowing better perfusion

COMPARATIVE MODES OF DELIVERY (% perinatal mortality)

SVD – 35.5%; LFD – 0%; MFD – 33.3%; VE – 33.3%; assisted breech extraction – 25%; total breech extraction or version and extraction – 10%; total of these – 26.9% compared to C-section – 3.4%

DERMATOLOGIC CONDITIONS COMMON TO OB/GYN

ACNE

Diagnosis

(1) Endocrine (PCO, Cushing's PMS, OCPs, etc.)?
(2) Seasonal changes?
(3) Exposure to heavy oils, etc?
(4) Occlusive or tight clothing, habits?
(5) Medications (corticosteroids, ACTH, androgens, danazol, iodides, bromides, INH, lithium, halothane, Vitamin B_{12}, cobalt radiation, hyperalimentation)?
(6) Fever and elevated WBC (acne fulminans)?
(7) Past treatments – broad-spectrum antibiotics – Gram-negative folliculitis (*Proteus, Pseudomonas*, or *Klebsiella* is grown out). Treat with Accutane or appropriate antibiotic
(8) Stress?

Treatment

(1) *Mild*
   (a) Benzoyl peroxide (Desquam-X or E, Benzac AC or W or Benzagel, Pan Oxyl)
   (b) Cleocin T solution 30 or 60 ml
   (c) Erythromycin base (Staticin, 60 ml; Eryderm, 60 ml; Erycette, T-stat pads)
(2) *Moderate*
   (a) Tretinoin (Retin A) q. hr on dry face or q.o.d.
      Use 0.025% cream or 0.01% gel for fair complexion
      Use 0.05% cream or 0.025% gel for others
      (cream preferred for dry skin; gel for oily skin)
   (b) Benzoyl peroxide at different time than Retin-A
(3) *Severe*
   (a) Tetracycline 500 mg b.i.d. on empty stomach. Decrease dose to 250–500 mg daily after lesions clear or increase dose after 4–6 wks to 2 g daily for several weeks if lesions have not subsided
   (b) Erythromycin 1 g daily effective
   (c) Minocycline, doxycycline
   (d) Ampicillin if pregnant
   *Warn patients about decreased effectiveness of OCs and dangers of sunlight (especially with doxycycline). Also consider sebaceous gland suppression
      Estrogens (Desogen, OrthoCept, Ortho Cyclen, Ovcon 35, Demulen, Brevicon, or Modicon)
      Prednisones (5–7.5 mg) q. hr
      Spironolactone 100–200 mg with meals. Monitor electrolytes

ROSACEA

Diagnosis

(1) Red flush of central face, neck, nose
(2) Rule out malignant carcinoid, lupus; basal cell carcinoma if rhinophyma present

Treatment

(1) Avoid hot food and drinks
(2) Tetracycline 500 mg p.o. b.i.d.
(3) Metrogel 0.75% x9 wks

HIDRADENITIS

Diagnosis

Large cysts, abscesses, in axilla, under breasts, groin, buttocks, anogenital region, thighs

Treatment

Antibiotics, prednisone, Accutane, surgery

MELASMA

Diagnosis

(1) Brown, macular facial pigmentation – increased with sun exposure (develops in 50–70% pregnant women)
(2) Common with OCs (5–34%)

Treatment

(1) Melanex 3%; Solaquin forte 4% b.i.d.
(2) Retin-A cream if not pregnant
(3) Avoid sun or use sun blocks
(4) Chemical peels

COWDEN'S DISEASE

Diagnosis

(1) Flesh, pink, or brown papules at midfacial, perioral, lips, ears
(2) Punctate keratoses of the palms and soles

Treatment

Assess for breast cancer (20%) – often bilateral
(1) Prophylactic mastectomy advocated
(2) Thyroid cancer (8%)

ALOPECIA

Diagnosis

(1) Drugs
(2) 2° Syphilis (moth-eaten appearance)
(3) Tinea capitis
(4) Androgenetic (androgen producing tumor?)

Treatment

Determine etiology – treat accordingly

SEBORRHEIC KERATOSIS

Diagnosis

(1)   Barely elevated small papule
(2)   Benign

Treatment

(1)   Electrocautery
(2)   Shave excision
(3)   Liquid nitrogen

DERMATOFIBROMAS

Diagnosis

(1)   Firm scar-like papules <1 cm
(2)   Usually on lower legs
(3)   If multiple, have been associated with lupus

Treatment

(1)   None
(2)   Excision
(3)   Cryotherapy

EYELID DERMATITIS

Diagnosis

(1)   Pruritic eruption of the periorbital ski
(2)   Common irritants: eye cosmetics, fragrance, preservatives, hair spray, nail polish

Treatment

(1)   D/c all products around eye, perfumes and nail polish
(2)   Use only unscented products on the facial area
(3)   Vaseline petroleum jelly or bland emollient as moisturizer
(4)   1–2.5% hydrocortisone cream, sparingly
(5)   Once clear for 7–10 days, add back one product at a time every 5 days
(6)   Consider patch testing p.r.n.

FUNGUS (toenails and/or fingernails)

Diagnosis

(1)   Trauma predisposes nail plate
(2)   Establish diagnosis with KOH prep. Fax (216) 844-1076 for Derm Pak

Treatment

(1)   Diflucan 150 mg weekly
(2)   Itraconazole (Sporanox) 200 mg/day. (Pulse dose with 400 mg/daily x first week of each month for 16 wks)
(3)   Lamisil 250 mg daily p.o. continous (6 wks for F.N.; 12 wks for T.N.)

POLYMORPHOLOGICAL URTICARIAL PAPULES OF PREGNANCY (PUPP)*

Diagnosis

(1) **Most common** in primigravida
(2) Usually >28 wks
(3) Increased with multiple births or increased weight gain
(4) Extreme pruritus starts on abdomen in striae
(5) **No risk** to infant or mother
(6) Resolves 2 wks postpartum (**seldom recurs**)

Treatment

(1) Aveeno baths
(2) Cool compresses
(3) Benadryl 25 mg p.o. q. 4–6 hrs
(4) Prednisone, phototherapy – deliver baby

HERPES GESTATIONIS*

Diagnosis

(1) **Rare** (1:50,000 pregnancies)
(2) *Not* associated with herpes virus despite name
(3) Eruption often starts periumbilical
(4) Usually 2nd or 3rd trimester
(5) **May recur** in subsequent pregnancies or with OCP use (usually earlier and more severe in subsequent pregnancies)
(6) Urticarial plaques with tense vesicles or bullae
(7) Fetal **risk unclear**
(8) Has been associated with trophoblastic disease

Treatment

Systemic and topical steroids

PRURITUS GRAVIDARUM*

Diagnosis

(1) Intense itching during pregnancy (usually more intense on extremities than trunk)
(2) Associated with cholestasis (itching associated with bile acids)
(3) Increase in infant mortality and prematurity
(4) **Usually recurs**
(5) **Most common** (1–2% pregnancies)

Treatment

(1) Topical steroids
(2) Oral Benadryl
(3) Cholestyramine

*Pregnancy specific dermatoses

ERYTHEMA NODOSUM

Diagnosis

(1) Tender, red nodules on lower extremities, especially shin
(2) Non-ulcerating
(3) Infections: TB, β hemolytic strep, lymphogranuloma venereum, *Yersinia*
(4) Systemic disease: pregnancy, ulcerative colitis
(5) Drugs: sulfonamides, oral contraceptives

PSORIASIS

Diagnosis

(1) Rich red hue, smooth plaque; genetic 1–3% – can occur at site of trauma
(2) Scaly, red follicular papules merge to form large, bright plaques
(3) Avoid lithium, beta-blockers, antimalarials, and systemic steroids

Treatment

(1) Betamethasone dipropionate (Diprotene, Alphatrex)
(2) Anthra-Derm 0.1, 0.25, 0.5, 1% ointment 1.5 oz., 42.5 g tubes
(3) Drithrocreme HP 1% Cream, 50 g tube
(4) PsoriGel 7.5% coal tar solution; 1% Alcohol Gel, 4 oz
(5) Topical steroids (pulse dosing – 2 wks of medication and 1 wk of lab only with plastic occlusion very effective) for psoriasis on <20% of body
(6) For more than 20% of body – consider dermatology referral for UVB/tar, PUVA, methotrexate, hydrea, etretinate, etc.

LICHEN SCLEROSUS

Diagnosis

(1) White "plaque-like" lesions, or leukoplakia of the vulva and/or perineum
(2) Biopsy necessary to rule out squamous carcinoma

Treatment

Clobetasol (Temovate) 0.05% cream or ointment (30 g)
For LSA, 12 week application with taper to 2x/wk combined with 1% hydrocortisone
For LSC, twice daily applications x10–14 days, 1% hydrocortisone. Monitor these patients closely every 6 months for squamous carcinoma

ATONIC DERMATITIS

Diagnosis

(1) Psitoris alba – on face
(2) Keratosis psitoris (goose skin) – on lateral thighs, upper arms

Treatment

(1) Steroids – ointments not creams
(2) Moisturize – eucerin cream or acetophil
(3) **No** Ivory or Dial soap

DERMATOLOGIC CONDITIONS COMMON TO OB/GYN

ANTIFUNGAL TREATMENT REGIMENS (TOPICAL)

(Source: official package inserts)
. As with all therapies, the diagnosis should be reviewed if no clinical improvement
occurs after prescribed treatment and appropriate follow-up

Topical antifungal	Tinea pedis	Tinea cruris/tinea corporis
Rx		
Lamisil* Cream, 1%[†] (terbinafine hydrochloride cream)	1–4 wks b.i.d.	1–4 wks q.d. or b.i.d.
Lotrisone* (clotrimazole/betametasone)	4 wks b.i.d.	2 wks b.i.d.
Loprox* (ciclopirox olamine)	4 wks b.i.d.	4 wks b.i.d.
Spectazole* (econazole nitrate)	4 wks b.i.d.	2 wks q.d.
Nizoral* (ketoconazole)	6 wks q.d.	2 wks q.d.
Monistat-Derm* (miconazole nitrate 2%)	4 wks b.i.d.	2 wks b.i.d.
Naftin* (naftifine hydrochloride)	4 wks q.d.	4 wks q.d.
Exelderm* (sulconazole nitrate)	4 wks b.i.d.	3 wks q.d. or b.i.d.
Oxistat* (oxiconazole nitrate)	4 wks q.d.	2 wks q.d.
OTC		
Tinactin* (tolnaftate)	4 wks b.i.d.	2 wks b.i.d. – tinea cruris 4 wks b.i.d. – tinea corporis
Micatin* (miconazole nitrate)	4 wks b.i.d.	2 wks b.i.d. – tinea cruris 4 wks b.i.d. – tinea corporis
Lotrimin AF* (clotrimazole)	4 wks b.i.d.	2 wks b.i.d. – tinea cruris 4 wks b.i.d. – tinea corporis
Desenex* (undecylenic acid and zinc undecylenate)	4 wks b.i.d.	Not indicated in package labeling
Cruex* (undecylenic acid and zinc undecylenate)	Not indicated in package labeling	2 wks b.i.d. – tinea cruris Not indicated in package labeling for tinea corporis

*Registered trademarks; [†]Lamisil Solution, 1% 30 ml spray bottle (tinea versicolor)

OTHER ANTIFUNGAL TREATMENT REGIMENS

Terazol-7 Cream   Use nightly x7 nights

Terazol-3 Suppository   Use nightly x3 nights

Vagistat   Use at night

Boric Acid   Vaginal suppositories 600 mg at night x2 wks

Ketoconazole   200 mg twice daily and then daily x5 days; OR twice daily x5 days (obtain liver panel prior to calling this in)

Nystatin   100,000 units oral, 60 ml bottle. 5 ml p.o. 4x day

DIABETES AND PREGNANCY

BACKGROUND

    (1)   2–3% pregnancies affected
    (2)   90% of this 2–3% represent GDM
    (3)   50% of women who develop GDM will develop overt DM within 20 years
    (4)   Women with overt DM who conceive have a 10-fold increase in maternal mortality and perinatal mortality of 4%

CLASSIFICATION

    A1   Diet-controlled GDM
    A2   GDM complicated by insulin use, hypertension, polyhydramnios, macrosomia, or prior stillbirth
    B   Overt; onset > age 20 and duration <10 years
    C   DM overt; onset age 10–19 or duration 10–19 years
    D   Juvenile onset or duration of 20 years or more
    F   Associated with nephropathy
    R   Associated with retinopathy
    T   Renal transplant patients

MAJOR MALFORMATIONS

    (1)   Increased x4
    (2)   Risks increased by 30% between 5–9 wks (embryogenesis)
    (3)   Spontaneous abortions increased by 35%
    (4)   Common: CNS, cardiac, renal, retinal
    (5)   Uncommon: caudal regression syndrome

SCREENING

    (1)   HbA1C: Preconception level (normal–similar to non-DM women)
                         Used to assess anomaly risk and to provide a goal for the woman aspiring to improve her chances of a good outcome
    (2)   Screen all women over 25 years of age at 24–28 wks
    (3)   Screen early in pregnancy (1st visit) and 24–28 wks those women with:
        (a)   Family history of DM
        (b)   Prior infant with cardiac anomaly
        (c)   History of stillbirth
        (d)   History of repeated pregnancy loss
        (e)   Previous child >4000 g

DIAGNOSIS

(1) If 1 hr 50-g p.o. glucose challenge test is >140 mg/dl
(2) 3 hr GTT of 100-g p.o. glucose after 3 days of adequate carb. intake. Two abnormal values are necessary to make diagnosis of GDM

Time	Glucose level (mg/dl)	
	WHO	*Carpenter & Coustan*
Fasting	<105	<95
1 hr	<190	<180
2 hrs	<165	<155
3 hrs	<145	<140

(3) If 1 hr 50-g test is greater

MANAGEMENT

(1) Goals: maintain FBS of 60–80 mg/dl; 2 hr pp levels of 60–100 mg/dl
(2) Diet: 2200–2400 kcal for women of normal weight
(3) Insulin: abdominal to achieve consistency and rotation and at perpendicular to skin to prevent intradermal injection rather than subq

NPH alone		*NPH + REG*			
AM	2/3	AM	2/3 – 2/3 NPH	1/3	REG
PM	1/3	PM	1/3 – 1/2 NPH (q.h.s.)	1/2	REG (AC)

SURVEILLANCE

(1) *Patient diary* (charting of glucose levels, insulin dosage, and date/time)
(2) *Type A1*: no amnio; delivery by 40 wks
(3) *Type A2, B, C*: twice weekly NSTs >34 wks; delivery at 38 wks if glucose levels abnl and PG present
(4) *Type D, F, R*: twice weekly NSTs from 28–30 wks; delivery at 36 wks if abnl glucose levels and PG present
(5) *Ultrasound* (fetal anatomy) with echocardiogram (serious consideration) 18–20 wks

PRE-TERM LABOR

(1) $MgSO_4$ or calcium channel blocker. (Avoid terbutaline if possible – tendency to cause hyperglycemia)
(2) Corticosteroids (for lung maturity, but know that hyperglycemia will probably result)

LABOR & DELIVERY

(1) Insulin (regular insulin 50 units in 500 ml NS)
     Shake well; run out 50 ml waste to ensure absorption of surfaces
     Continuous pump rate of 0.5 units/hr or > with increments of 0.5–1 unit/hr to obtain necessary glucose levels
(2) D5LR
(3) Bedside glucose values every hour with finger stick test strips
(4) Adjust infusion p.r.n. to maintain glucose levels 100–130 mg/dl

DIABETES AND PREGNANCY

DIABETES-IN-PREGNANCY PROGRAM PROTOCOL

CLASS A AND A/B
- (1) Glucose determination weekly
- (2) Biweekly visits until 34 wks, then weekly
- (3) Ultrasound examination every month
- (4) Non-stress test at 34 wks, then weekly
- (5) HbA-1C not necessary
- (6) No 24-hr urine, ophthalmologic evaluation, or fetal ECG necessary
- (7) Daily fetal movement counts

CLASS B AND C
- (1) Daily home glucose monitoring
- (2) Biweekly visits until 34 wks, then weekly
- (3) Ultrasound: dating at 20 wks (profile and echocardiogram), then monthly
- (4) HbA-1C monthly
- (5) Non-stress test at 33 wks, then weekly
- (6) Ophthalmologic evaluation, follow-up according to findings
- (7) 24-hr urine initially and in each trimester
- (8) Daily fetal movement counts

CLASS D TO H
Above, plus the following: ECG initially, uric acid, liver function tests, fibrinogen, and fibrin split products in each trimester

DELIVERY TIME
Class A and B: <42 weeks' gestation
Class C to H: at term gestation or pulmonic maturity (weekly amniocentesis starting at 38.5 wks)

LABOR
- (1) Blood glucose to be maintained at <100 mg/dl
- (2) Intravenous: D5 ½ nl saline solution and 10 units of regular insulin ml/hr – 1 unit insulin/hr
- (3) D5 ½ nl saline solution piggy-backed to insulin-carry solution to adjust glycemia
- (4) Hourly finger-stick blood glucose determinations

DIABETES AND PREGNANCY

DIABETES SCREENING

50-g oral glucose load, between 24 and 28 weeks' gestation, without regard to time of day or prandial state; venous plasma glucose measured 1 hr later
If value ≥140 mg/dl – schedule 3-hr GTT

3-HR GTT

100-g oral glucose load in a.m. > fast of 8 hrs
Patient should remain seated and not smoke throughout testing
    FBS ≥105
    1 hr ≥190
    2 hr ≥165
    3 hr ≥145

If screen is normal, no further dipstick required after 24 weeks' gestation (for glucosuria) (*Green J* 1995;86:number 3 (Sept))

ABNL GTT (CLASS A + B) [IF 3 HR GTT ABNL]

Glucose weekly
Biweekly visits until 34 wks, then weekly
Ultrasound every month
NST at 34 wks, then weekly
Daily fetal movement counts

DIABETES AND PREGNANCY

ANTEPARTUM SURVEILLANCE OF THE DIABETIC PREGNANCY

Test	When to initiate
Maternal assessment of fetal activity	28 wks
Non-stress test	Weekly beginning at 28 wks; twice wkly beginning at 34 wks
Contraction stress test	Any time a nonreactive non-stress test is obtained

Biophysical profile
  Non-stress test
  Fetal body movements
  Fetal breathing
  Fetal tone
  Volume of amniotic fluid
	In conjunction with contraction stress test

Hemoglobin A1C levels	Early in gestation or upon presentation for prenatal care, also at any time maternal compliance is questioned
Ultrasound	Every 4–6 wks (to screen for fetal macrosomia, fetal size, and determination of the best route for delivery)

DIABETES AND PREGNANCY

PATIENT-MONITORED CAPILLARY BLOOD GLUCOSE GOALS DURING PREGNANCY IN DIABETIC WOMEN

Specimen	Blood glucose (mg/dl)
Fasting	60–90 (3.3–5.0 mM)
Pre-meal	60–105 (3.3–5.8 mM)
Postprandial 1 hr	100–120 (5.5–6.7 mM)
0200–0600	60–120 (3.3–6.7 mM)

RISK FACTORS FOR GESTATIONAL DIABETES

- Age 30 or older
- Obesity
- Hypertension
- Glycosuria during the current pregnancy
- Prior delivery of an infant with birth weight >9 lbs
- Prior stillbirth
- One or more family members with diabetes mellitus

DIABETES AND PREGNANCY

SCREENING AND DIAGNOSTIC CRITERIA FOR GESTATIONAL DIABETES MELLITUS

Screening

All pregnant women without a diagnosis of gestational diabetes prior to 24 wks;

50-g oral glucose load, between 24 and 28 weeks' gestation, without regard to time of day or prandial state;
venous plasma glucose measured 1 hr later; and

Value of ≥140 mg/dl (7.8 mmol/l in venous plasma indicates need for 3-hr glucose test)

Diagnosis

100-g oral glucose load, administered in morning after overnight fast of 8–14 hrs and after at least 3 days of unrestricted diet (≥150 g carbohydrate) and physical activity;

Venous plasma glucose is measured at fasting, 1, 2, and 3 hrs after glucose load (subject should remain seated and not smoke throughout test; and

Two or more of the following venous plasma concentrations must be met or exceeded for positive diagnosis:

Fasting	105 mg/dl (5.8 mmol/l)
1 hr	190 mg/dl (10.6 mmol/l)
2 hr	165 mg/dl (9.2 mmol/l)
3 hr	145 mg/dl (8.1 mmol/l)

American College of Obstetricians & Gynecologists (1994) criteria for diagnosis of gestational diabetes using 100 g glucose taken orally – gestational diabetes is diagnosed when any two values are met or exceeded

Timing of measurement	*Plasma glucose* (mg/dl)	
	National Diabetes Data Group (1979)	*Carpenter & Coustan (1982)*
Fasting	<105	<95
1 hr	<190	<180
2 hr	<165	<155
3 hr	<145	<140

DIABETES AND PREGNANCY

CLASSIFICATION OF DIABETES COMPLICATING PREGNANCY

Class	Onset	Fasting plasma glucose	2-hr Postprandial glucose	Therapy
A1	Gestational	<105 mg/dl	<120 mg/dl	Diet
A2	Gestational	>105 mg/dl	>120 mg/dl	Insulin

Class	Age/onset	Duration (yrs)	Vascular disease	Therapy
B	Over 20	<10	None	Insulin
C	10 to 19	10 to 19	None	Insulin
D	Before 10	>20	Benign retinopathy	Insulin
F	Any	Any	Nephropathy*	Insulin
R	Any	Any	Proliferative retinopathy	Insulin
H	Any	Any	Heart	Insulin

*When diagnosed during pregnancy: 500 mg or more proteinuria per 24 hrs measured before 20 weeks' gestation

DIABETES AND PREGNANCY

CLASSIFICATION OF DIABETES IN PREGNANCY

Pre-gestational diabetes

Class	Age of onset (yrs)	Duration (yrs)	Vascular disease	Therapy
A	Any	Any	No	Diet only
B	>20	<10	No	Insulin
C	10–19	10–19	No	Insulin
D	Before 10	>20	Benign retinopathy	Insulin
F	Any	Any	Nephropathy	Insulin
R	Any	Any	Proliferative retinopathy	Insulin
H	Any	Any	Heart disease	Insulin

Gestational diabetes

Class	Fasting glucose level	Postprandial glucose level
A_1	<105 mg/dl and	<120 mg/dl
A_2	>105 mg/dl and/or	>120 mg/dl

DIABETES AND PREGNANCY

GESTATIONAL DIABETES

Screening

(50-g glucose, check glucose 1 hr later; if >135, 3 hr GTT)
- (1) First visit and at 28 wks for patients with one of the following risk factors:
    - (a) Family hx of DM   (*H/o repeated pregnancy loss)
    - (b) >25% above IBW   (*Previous child >4000 g)
- (2) All other OB patients: 24–28 wks

Diagnosis

- (1) All patients with abnl 1hr *or* random glucose >135
- (2) 3 hr GTT
    - (a) Nl activity
    - (b) No intercurrent illness
    - (c) Adequate diet for 3 days prior to test
    - (d) Fasting glucose – 100 g glucose – blood glucose at 1 hr, 2 hrs, 3 hrs

ABNORMAL VALUES*:		
FBS	>105	
1-hr	>190	*Two or more = GDM
2-hr	>165	
3-hr	>145	

Management

- (1) Diet modification
    - (a) Consult nutritionist *or*
    - (b) 36 kcal/kg or 15 kcal/lb(IBW) + 100 kcal/trimester
    - (c) Diet composition: 40–50% CHO, 12–20% protein, 30–35% fat
- (2) Glucose monitoring (Pt diary)
    - (a) FBS <105, 2-hr post-prandial <120 q.d.
    - (b) If either consistently abnl, insulin

Insulin

Anticipated requirements:

EGA			
	6–18 wks	0.7 U/kg	Type I & II DM (pre-existing)
	18–26 wks	0.8 U/kg	Type I & II DM (pre-existing)
	26–36 wks	0.9 U/kg	
	36–40 wks	1.0 U/kg	

Initiate therapy at ½ above doses

Distribution

NPH alone	*NPH + REG*	
AM 2/3	AM 2/3 – 2/3 NPH	1/3 REG
PM 1/3	PM 1/3 – 1/2 NPH(qHS)	1/2 REG (AC)

Change only one insulin dose per week

Pt diary AC & HS (8, 12, 17, 22)

DIABETES AND PREGNANCY

MATERNAL/FETAL SURVEILLANCE

Type I/II IDDM

Mother (at intake)
   – thyroid panel, 24-hr urine protein/Cr Cl/BUN/Ophtho consult/HgA,C (then q. 6 wks)
Fetus   – NST protocol

– mother with vascular disease	30–33 wk	q. wk
	34–36 wk	3 x per wk
	36+ wk	q. d
– no vascular disease	32–35 wk	q. wk
	36–37 wk	3 x per wk
	37+ wk	q. d

Gestational DM

Maternal – HA,C q. 6 wks
Fetus   – NST protocol

– diet-controlled	38+ wk	q. wk
– insulin requiring	32–35 wk	q. wk
(same as above; no vasc dx)	36–37 wk	3 x per wk
	37+wk	q. d

Consider AOC after 36 wks for FLM in insulin-requiring

PROBLEMS WHEN DIABETES IS A FACTOR

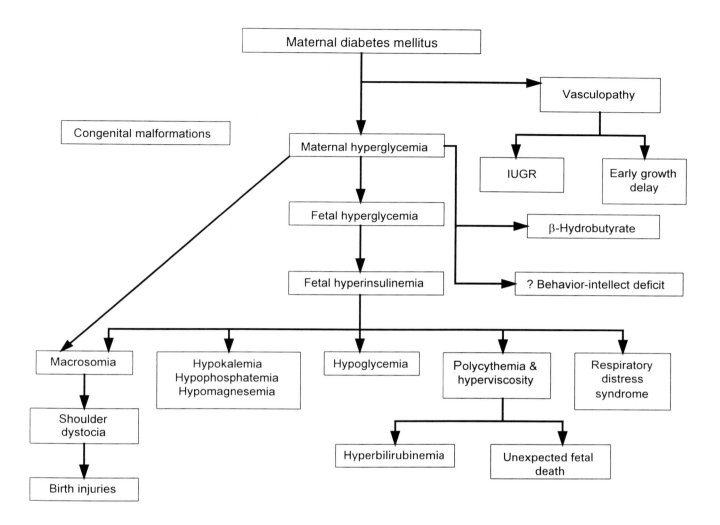

DYSTOCIA

PREDICT SHOULDER DYSTOCIA

Mid-pelvic delivery
Prolonged 2nd stage   ↑ 23%
Macrosomia

Macrosomia
(>4.5 kg)   ↑ 50%
Diabetes

Should be fully appraised of options

1000s of C/S's + the risks, complications, morbidity and mortality are needed to prevent just a few dystocia cases – (ileus, hemorrhage, P.E.)

RISKS

		Weight (g)	%Dystocia
(1)	>8#	<3000	0.2
		3000–3499	0.8
		3500–3999	2.3–2.9
		4000–4499	8.6–10.3
		>4500	24–35.7

(2)   Antepartum
      (a)   Birth weight
      (b)   Fundal height
      (c)   Maternal diabetes
      (d)   Maternal pre-pregnancy weight; maternal wt gain during pregnancy
      (e)   Post-term pregnancy (>42 wks)
      (f)   Prior delivery with shoulder dystocia
      (g)   Wt of largest previous infant (>4500 g)

(3)   Intrapartum
      (a)   Prolonged second stage
      (b)   Prolonged second stage plus mid-pelvic delivery
      (c)   Prolonged decel phase

MANAGEMENT

Maneuvers of shoulder dystocia
(Initially call for help if available)

      (1)   McRobert's
      (2)   Suprapubic pressure
      (3)   Wood's maneuver – corkscrew
          Post-shoulder 180 degrees. Body not head – not independent of body
      (4)   Mazzanti maneuver
          Delivery of post-shoulder; trace humerus to elbow, flex elbow so forearm is first delivered across chest and out

(5)   Fractures
      (a)   Clavicle
      (b)   Humerus
(6)   Extended episiotomy – 4th degree procto episiotomy

NEVER APPLY EXCESSIVE TRACTION

(7)   Zavanelli maneuver
      Cephalic replacement as initial maneuver rather than last resort if difficulty encountered
      especially to those that are inexperienced in dystocia treatment
      (*Green J* 1993;82: number 5 (Nov))
      Some sources say try to avoid at all cost secondary to increase neurological injuries and
      decreased experience. (@ 40 known documented cases)
(8)   Mueller Hillis maneuver
      (*Green J* 1993;82:number 4, Ptl; (Oct))
      Applying fundal pressure to see if head moves down in pelvis – not recommended anymore

Brachial plexus injury

Erb's C_{5-6}

Klumpke's C_8-T_1

Some are spontaneous

Some are encountered without chart documentation
      3–5%   <4.5kg
      15–30%   >4.5kg

80% resolve in 1 year. The remainder usually show partial recovery without surgery – others
unfortunately –
      Asphyxia: 20% noted in surviving infants of dystocia. 5–10 min from time cord compressed
      Fractured humerus or clavicle – minor – resolve

ECTOPIC PREGNANCY

EXCLUSION CRITERIA FOR MEDICAL MANAGEMENT

Active pulmonary disease

Adnexal mass >3.5 cm

Aspartate transaminase >50 IU/l

Creatinine >1.3 mg/dl

Extrauterine gestation + cardiac activity

Free fluid + pelvic pain

Hemodynamic instability

Patient noncompliance

White blood cell <3000/mm^3

ECTOPIC PREGNANCY

NON-SURGICAL MANAGEMENT

DX:

(1)   hCG if <50% increase in 48 hrs then abn pregnancy
(2)   If hCG >2000 and with intrauterine GS then abnl pregnancy consider ectopic
(3)   If dx abnl pregnancy; if hCG rises or falls very slowly and no POC or path – strong suspicion ectopic

Serum progesterone: <5 ng/ml   Abnl pregnancy
                             >25 ng/ml   Viable pregnancy
                             Most ectopic   Prog <15 ng/ml

Single dose methotrexate – dose – 50 mg/m^2 IM

Inclusion criteria: hCG rising, hemodynamically stable
                        Transvaginal sono – unruptured ectopic
                        Ectopic mass <3.5cm
                        Patient desires future fertility

Exclusion criteria: Declining hCG after D&C
                        Mass >3.5 cm
                        Hemodynamically unstable
                        Desires sterilization
                        Previous sterilization
                        Abnl CBC or SGOT

Patient instructions: No alcohol
                        No intercourse
                        No vitamins or folic acid
                        Contraception

Protocol & F/u: Day 0:   hCG, D&C (?), CBC with diff, SGOT, creatinine
                        Day 1:   hCG, methotrexate
                        Day 4:   hCG
                        Day 7:   hCG

hCG on Day #7 should be 15% less than Day 4. If not, repeat MTX. If cardiac activity on EV, repeat EV qod until no cardiac activity

Usually have increased pain post MTX injection

If pain increased, check Hct. If lower than previous MTX, do sonogram for increased fluid in cul-de-sac

Most hCG titers D4 > D1

Meantime to resolution 35–40 days; for hCG to be <5

5.8% failure rate

14.3% failure rate if cardiac activity seen

83% tubal patency rate post-resolution by HSG

Recurrent ectopic rate < linear salpingotomy

ECTOPIC PREGNANCY

METHOTREXATE THERAPY FOR PERSISTENT ECTOPIC PREGNANCY

Route	Dosage	Success number (%)
Oral	10 mg p.o. q.d. x5 days	1/1 (100%)
		2/2 (100%)
		1/1 (100%)
	5 mg p.o. q.d. x5 days	1/1 (100%)
	5–10 mg p.o. q.d. x5–7 days	14/15 (94%)
IV	100 mg/m^2 IV bolus over 1 hr, then 200 mg/m^2 IV over 12 hr, leucovorin 10 mg/m^2 p.o. q. 12 hr x4 doses	3/3 (100%)
IM	1 mg/kg IM q.o.d. x3 doses Alternating leucovorin 0.1 mg/kg IM q.o.d. x3 doses	1/1 (100%)
	50 mg/m^2 IM x1 dose, No leucovorin	19/19 (100%)
Local	Not evaluated	

ECTOPIC PREGNANCY
Patient at risk (before 6 weeks)

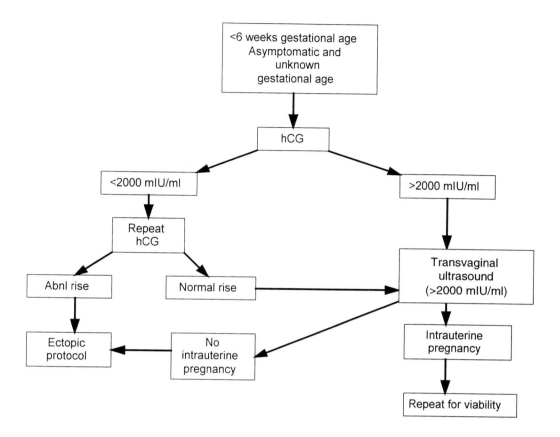

ECTOPIC PREGNANCY
Patient at risk (after 6 weeks)

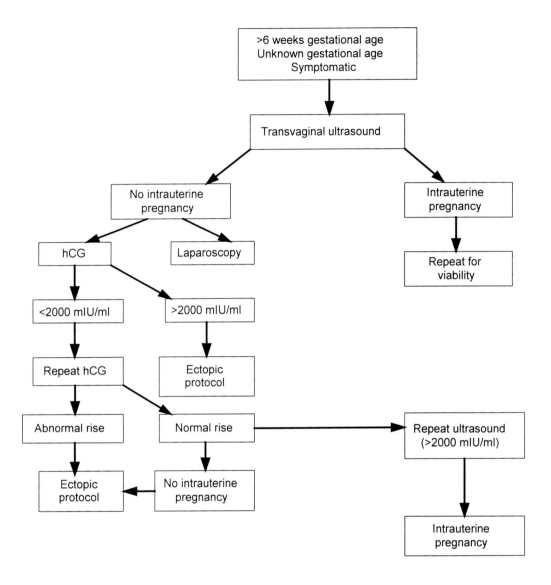

ECTOPIC PROTOCOL

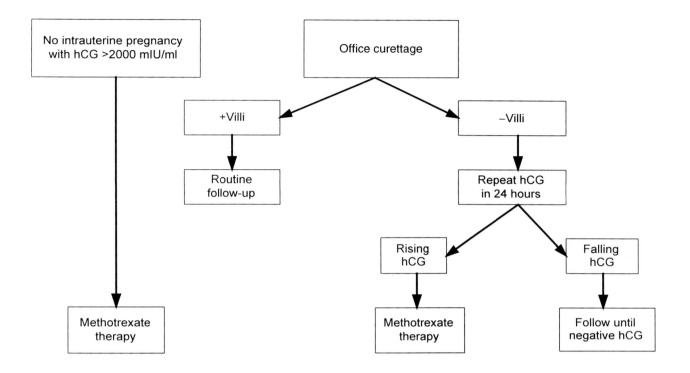

ECTOPIC PREGNANCY

Female patient with lower abdominal pain or abnormal bleeding

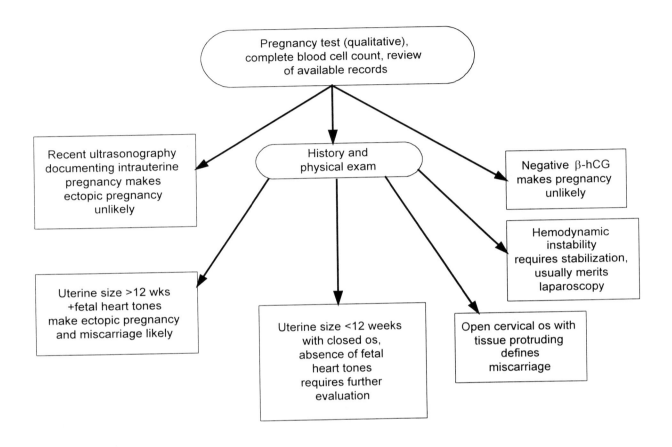

Pregnancy test (qualitative), complete blood cell count, review of available records

Recent ultrasonography documenting intrauterine pregnancy makes ectopic pregnancy unlikely

History and physical exam

Negative β-hCG makes pregnancy unlikely

Hemodynamic instability requires stabilization, usually merits laparoscopy

Uterine size >12 wks +fetal heart tones make ectopic pregnancy and miscarriage likely

Uterine size <12 weeks with closed os, absence of fetal heart tones requires further evaluation

Open cervical os with tissue protruding defines miscarriage

ECTOPIC PREGNANCY

**Pregnant patient with lower abdominal pain or abnormal
bleeding, uterine size <12 weeks or no fetal heart tones,
cervical os closed, hemodynamically stable**

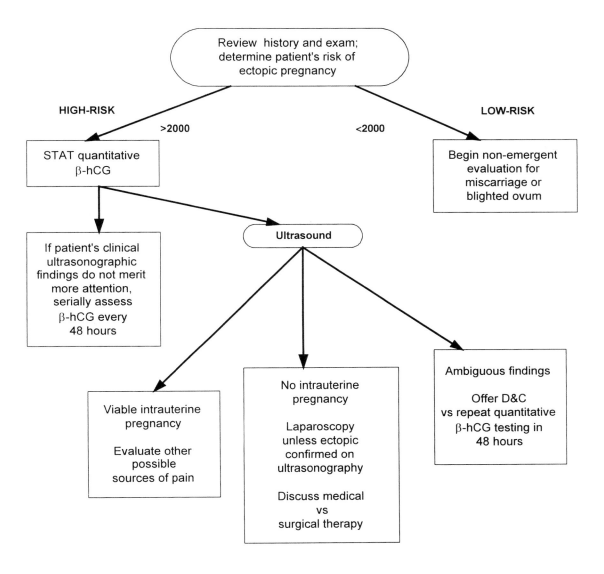

Risk factors include history of STDs or PID, ectopic pregnancy, pelvic surgery, or prior IUD use; signs of peritoneal irritation (e.g. guarding, rebound); hemodynamic instability; and unreliable or noncompliant patient

ENDOMETRIAL BIOPSY

INTERPRETING THE ENDOMETRIAL BIOPSY

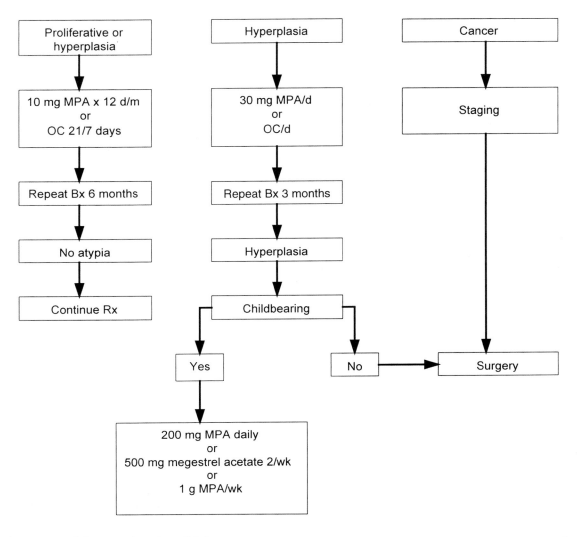

Atypia increases risk toward endometrial cancer

Remember: 'penny, nickel, dime and quarter'

Penny: simple hyperplasia 1%

Nickel: complex hyperplasia without atypia 5%

Dime: simple hyperplasia with atypia 10%

Quarter: complex hyperplasia with atypia 25–30%

ENDOMETRITIS

Signs and symptoms suggesting postpartum endometritis are fever greater than 100.4 °F (38 °C) within 36 hrs of delivery, malaise, tachycardia, lower abdominal pain and tenderness, uterine tenderness and malodorous lochia.

Endometritis is a polymicrobial infection caused by microorganisms that are part of the normal vagina flora. These bacteria gain access to the upper genital tract, peritoneal cavity, and occasionally, the bloodstream as a result of vaginal examinations during labor and manipulation during surgery.

The most common pathogenic bacteria are group B streptococci, anaerobic streptococci, aerobic Gram-negative bacilli (predominantly *E. coli*, *K. pneumoniae* and *Proteus* species) and anaerobic Gram-negative bacilli (principally *Bacteroides* and *Prevotella* species).

The principal risk factors for endometritis are:
(1)   Cesarean delivery – 30–35% if the C-section is performed after extended period of labor and ruptured membranes without antibiotic prophylaxis and 15–20% with prophylaxis
(2)   Young age
(3)   Low socioeconomic status
(4)   Extended duration of labor and ruptured membranes
(5)   Multiple vaginal examinations

MANAGEMENT

Regimen #1:   Clindamycin 500 mg IV q. 8 hr
                Gentamicin 1.5 mg/kg IV q. 8 hr

Regimen #2:   Clindamycin 900 mg IV q. 8 hr
                Aztreonam 1–2 g IV q. 8 hr

Regimen #3:   Metronidazole 500 mg IV q. 6 hr
                Penicillin 5 mu IV q. 6 hr
                Ampicillin 2 g IV q. 6 hr
                Mefoxin 2 g IV q. 6 hr
                Unasyn 3 g IV stat then 1.5 g IV q. 6 hr

(1)   Patients who have mild to moderately severe infections, particularly after vaginal delivery, can be treated with short IV courses of single agents

(2)   Combination antibiotic regimens should be considered for more severely ill patients

(3)   Once antibiotics are begun, approximately 90% of patients will defervesce within 48–72 hrs. When the patient has been afebrile and asymptomatic for approximately 24 hrs, parenteral antibiotics should be discontinued and the patient discharged

(4)   If the patient's fever persists despite apparently appropriate antimicrobial therapy, search for a hidden abscess by bimanual examination or pelvic ultrasound and careful check of the abdominal wound

(5)   Patients who remain febrile with hectic fever spikes and in whom an abscess has been ruled out must be evaluated for the possibility of septic pelvic thrombophlebitis. Treatment with full intravenous heparin anticoagulation will usually result in rapid lysis of the fever within 48 hrs

EPIDURAL ANALGESIA

DOSAGES

(1) Marcaine 0.75% (Bupivacaine)   20 cc
     Normal saline   30 cc
     Fentanyl 250 µg/5 ml (Sublimaze)   <u>10 cc</u>
                                         60 cc

Use test dose of 3 cc (epinephrine) solution. Then top off dose 3–6 cc followed by 6 cc/hr rate. Use this formula for expected long labors and less motor blockade.

(2) Lidocaine 2% with Epi (1:200,000)   20 cc
     8.4% Sodium bicarbonate (50 ml vial)   2 cc
     Fentanyl 100 µg/2 ml (Sublimaze)   <u>2 cc</u>
                                             24 cc

Use this solution for more of a sensory blockade for postpartum tubals, C-sections, and expected operative deliveries. Same dosages as above except C-sections then inject 3 cc test dose, slow 12 cc bolus and add 5 more cc if T10 level not reached after few minutes.

(3) Xylocaine 2% (10 ml vial x2)   20 cc
     8.4% Sodium bicarbonate (50 ml vial)   2 cc
     Fentanyl 100 µg/2 ml (Sublimaze)   <u>2 cc</u>
                                             24 cc

Use this formula in same type situations as in #2, but with the exception of patient having PIH or condition that contradicts the use of epinephrine.

For potential complications see pages 71–72

EPIDURAL ANALGESIA

POTENTIAL COMPLICATIONS

Complication	Incidence	Presumed etiology, signs or symptoms	Treatment
Maternal hypotension (most common)	Approx. 22%	Sympathetic blockade leading to vasodilatation, vascular pooling, diminished venous return	Volume preload with 500–1000 ml or balanced salt solution; left uterine displacement; avoid supine position; ephedrine if additional therapy required
Maternal central nervous (high spinal)	0.06%	Unintentional subarachnoid injection of local anesthetic; severe hypotension, profound bradycardia, respiratory compromise	Support airway; intubate; 100% O_2; intravenous fluids; vasopressors
Maternal central nervous system toxicity	0.03–0.5%	Intravascular injection of local anesthetic leading to slurred speech, dizziness, tinnitus, metallic taste, oral paresthesias, syncope, seizures, coma, potential cardiopulmonary arrest (bupivacaine cardiotoxicity)	Oxygenate; intubate if necessary; treat seizures with thiopental or diazepam; uterine displacement; IV fluids; vasopressors; CPR if needed
Maternal temperature elevation	Directly proportional to duration of epidural	Sympathetic nervous system blockade thought to inhibit heat loss	Antibiotics if intrauterine infection suspected (temp. usually $\geq 38\,^{\circ}C$)
Post-dural puncture headache	1–2%	Loss of cerebrospinal fluid (CSF) through puncture site with decreased CSF pressure. Onset several hours to days after puncture; headache on sitting or standing; relief when horizontal	Conservative: rest in horizontal position; hydrate; analgesics; caffeine; if no relief, epidural blood patch
Transient rise in fetal transcutaneous pCO_2	Unknown	May be associated with either decreased uteroplacental perfusion or maternal hyperventilation due to pain, anxiety	None necessary
Fetal abnormal heart rate pattern	Dependent on hypotension, maternal position, contraction pattern	Fall in maternal blood pressure leading to uteroplacental insufficiency; exacerbated by aortocaval compression or uterine hyperstimulation	Correction of hypotension by hydration; left uterine displacement; avoid supine position; avoid uterine hyperstimulation

71

EPIDURAL ANALGESIA

SOME NEUROLOGICAL COMPLICATIONS REPORTED WITH REGIONAL ANALGESIA

Cause		Lesion or event	Sequelae
Needle trauma during spinal or epidural		Nerve root lesion	Numbness and paresthesia
Vertebral stenosis		Nerve root lesion	
Epidural hematoma, abscess, or tumor		Space-occupying lesion Nerve root lesion	
Coagulopathy		Space-occupying lesion Nerve root lesion	
Vasculitis Hypotension Epinephrine		Cord ischemia	Paralysis, anterior spinal artery syndrome
Infection		Chronic arachnoiditis	Low back pain, cauda equina syndrome
Error	Wrong agent	Pentothal, phenol, iodine-containing skin disinfectant, radiographic contrast media, detergents	
	Wrong solution	Low pH or hypo-osmotic solution, preservatives and antioxidants from multidose vials resulting in cord ischemia or arachnoiditis	
	Wrong volume	Total spinal, spinal fluid leakage and displacement	Reversible total paralysis, headache, diplopia from paresis of IVth and VIth nerves

EPILEPSY

PRECONCEPTION

   (1)   Folic acid 4 mg daily x1 month prior to conception
   (2)   Compliance taking seizure meds important

       (a)   Risk of congenital malformations 2.4x greater than unaffected pts — inform pts
       (b)   Much worse if seizures occur causing hypoxia
       (c)   Most epileptic women have normal babies
       (d)   Try to decrease the number of seizure meds unless impossible to prevent seizures

   (3)   Inform and document risks to infant
       (a)   Coagulation disorders
       (b)   Craniofacial dysmorphic features
       (c)   Development delays
       (d)   Drug withdrawal problems
       (e)   Feeding difficulties
       (f)   Congenital anomalies (cleft lip and palate)
       (g)   Shortened fingers
       (h)   Seizures
       (i)   Increased perinatal problems (including increased incidence of stillbirths)

**The above are slightly increased over general population, but seizures can cause much worse problems so emphasize importance of staying on medication

ANTENATAL

   (1)   Obtain plasma anticonvulsant levels every 3–4 wks or more frequent if seizures, drug interaction, or toxicity develop
   (2)   Raise doses if necessary to maintain effective anticonvulsant activity. (Use 30 mg rather than 100 mg phenytoin capsules)
   (3)   If seizure control is not maintained and anticonvulsant dose has been increased until toxic effects are apparent, add additional anticonvulsant medication. Prescribe folic acid 1 mg and follow CBC (folic acid deficiency is common)

Early management

Rx nausea and vomiting early so patient able to take antiepileptic meds

Second trimester

MSAFP
Level II ultrasound
Review seizure frequency
Consider amniocentesis

Third trimester

Begin NST every week at 34 wks
Begin daily fetal kick count movements
Vitamin K therapy at 32 wks
       10 mg p.o. daily at 32–36 wks
       20 mg p.o. daily at 36 wks until delivery
       10 mg IV during labor

Postpartum

Decrease anticonvulsant meds. Check patient every 3–4 wks after delivery
Breast-feeding is not contraindicated while mother is on anticonvulsants

EXAMINATION SCHEDULE

Age	Complete physical*	Screening examinations	Screening tests	Immunizations
20–39	Every 5 yrs	Blood pressure annually	Pap smear every 1–3 years**	Diphtheria and tetanus every 10 yrs
		Breast every 1–3 yrs	Serum cholesterol every 5 yrs	Rubella once if necessary
		Pelvic every 1–3 yrs	Rubella titer at age 20	
			Mammography at age 35	
40–49	Every 3 yrs	Blood pressure annually	Pap smear every 1–3 yrs	Diphtheria and tetanus every 10 years
		Breast annually	Mammography every year	
		Pelvic annually	Occult blood every year	
			Serum cholesterol every 5 years	
			Tonometry	
50–69	Every 2 yrs	Blood pressure annually	Mammography annually	Influenza annually
		Breast annually	Occult blood annually	Pneumococcal vaccine at 65
		Pelvic annually	Pap smear every 3 yrs	Diphtheria and tetanus every 10 years
		Proctosigmoid-oscopy every 3 years	Serum cholesterol every 5 yrs	
			Tonometry every 2 yrs	
70 & up	Annually	Proctosigmoid-oscopy every 3 years	Mammography annually	Influenza annually
			Occult blood annually	
			Tonometry annually	

*Includes health risk and hearing assessment with education about exercise, nutrition, stress management, smoking, alcohol and drug abuse, seat belt use, repeated excessive exposure to the sun, and osteoporosis

**After two consecutive negative results

EXERCISE AND PREGNANCY

MAJOR QUESTIONS

   (1)   Increases in nonworking tissues produces vasoconstriction. (Does pregnant uterus have same vasomotor mechanism?)

   (2)   Increased body temperature – shift of blood volume from nonworking tissues (splanchnic + renal) to working tissues (muscle + skin)

RECOMMENDATIONS

   (1)   Mild to moderate exercise does not have to be curtailed during pregnancy

   (2)   Avoid hyperthermia. (Not in excess of 102 °F). Fetus is at 1 °C warmer than mother. Avoid more than 10 min in sauna or hot tub

   (3)   Avoid difficult activities (skiing or horseback riding) that require increased coordination secondary to increased productions of relaxins that cause increases in uncoordination and increases the chance of accident

   (4)   Decrease overall performance to about 50% of nonpregnant levels in third trimester

   (5)   Non-weight bearing exercise can be maintained at higher levels throughout pregnancy

   (6)   Avoid supine position during exercise after first trimester. (Decreases cardiac output in that position)

   (7)   Maintain adequate carbohydrate diet – avoid hypoglycemia

   (8)   Increase heat dissipation (appropriate hydration, clothing, and avoidance of adverse environmental conditions.)

RELATIVE CONTRAINDICATIONS TO EXERCISE

   (1)   Incompetent cervix

   (2)   Twins after 24 weeks' gestation
          Multiple gestation >24 wks or when fundal height is term

   (3)   History of PTL

   (4)   Known placenta previa after second trimester or if bleeding at any trimester

   (5)   PROM

   (6)   History of PIH

   (7)   Essential hypertension

   (8)   Certain cardiac diseases

   (9)   History of IUGR

   (10)   Cardiac arrhythmia

   (11)   Asthma or COPD

   (12)   Type II diabetes mellitus

   (13)   Breech presentation during third trimester

   (14)   Previous sedentary life-style

   (15)   Underweight

   (16)   Obesity

   (17)   Iron-deficiency anemia

   (18)   Recurrent spontaneous abortion of unknown origin (first trimester)

*Gravid patient should not get out of breath while exercising
*Formula: 70% of 220, minus woman's age. (Example: 30-yr-old pregnant woman should not extend her pulse rate >125 b.p.m.)
*High-risk pregnancies should avoid the stresses of excessive exercise and hyperthermia

EXERCISE PROGRAMS

    (1)   Squatting positions – decrease incidence of forceps and shorten secondary stage labor
    (2)   Pelvic floor exercises – may benefit postpartum for muscles to return to the pre-pregnancy condition
    (3)   Toning exercises – helps maintain proper posture and prevents lower back pain
    (4)   Semi-recumbent/sitting – not supine exercises to avoid aortocaval compression syndrome
    (5)   Recreational and sports activities – okay, but orthopedic risk
    (6)   Jogging – do not *initiate* after pregnancy. Limit to about 2 miles per day to prevent hyperthermia and dehydration. 4–6 mile brisk walk. Pay attention to terrain and wear shoes with proper support
    (7)   Aerobics – consistent with jogging recommendations
        (a)   Programs should have a scientific basis
        (b)   Avoid overextension + exercises on back
        (c)   Avoid hard surfaces and limit reps to 10
        (d)   Warm-up and cool-down should be done gradually

BICYCLING
    (1)   Program can be started during pregnancy
    (2)   Stationary cycle is preferable to standard bicycling because of weight and balance changes during pregnancy
    (3)   Bicycling should be avoided out of doors during high temperatures and high pollution levels

SWIMMING – may be the best
    (1)   Respiratory changes may make swimming difficult in late pregnancy
    (2)   Calisthenic exercise in water is encouraged for maintenance of strength and flexibility
    (3)   Avoid water that is too cold or too hot
    (4)   Jacuzzi temps >38.5 °C should be avoided

SCUBA DIVING – **avoid**
    Fetus may be at greater risk than mother (decompression sickness, hyperoxia, hypoxia, hypercapnia, and asphyxia)

MUSCULAR STRENGTH & ENDURANCE – increases chance of transient hypertension (Valsalva maneuver)
    (1)   Training with light weights can cautiously continue in pregnancy
    (2)   Avoid heavy resistance on weight machines
    (3)   Avoid use of heavy free weights. Use close spotter for light free weights
    (4)   Avoid Valsalva maneuver – use proper breathing

CONTACT SPORTS – avoid after first trimester

GROUP B BETA STREPTOCOCCUS

Group B Beta Strep is responsible for causing 15,000 cases of neonatal sepsis. The number of early-onset disease cases decreases with intrapartum prophylaxis for GBBS carriers. Although prophylaxis is widely accepted, there is still debate as to the best strategy for identifying women who are carriers. Also, cost-effective – necessity of antepartum screening has come under question.

Asymptomatic colonization GBBS is present in 15–40% of pregnant women. (Variation in colonization rate 2 degrees to ethnicity, geographic location, number sites cultured as well as methods of culture.)

> African Americans >21%; Hispanics 20.9%; Whites 13.7%;
> Hisp (Caribbean descent) 28%; (Mexican descent) 9.2%;
> Diabetics 2x higher – 20 vs 10%

Isolation rates highest from introitus, rectum, cervix

Supports concept gastrointestinal tract as reservoir

Vertical transmission occurs 40–73% of infants of colonized women

For every 100 colonized women, only 1 infant will develop GBBS

Overall, attack rate ranges from 1 to 3 per 1000 live births

RISK FACTORS FOR NEONATAL GBBS

> Preterm labor
> Preterm, PROM
> ROM >18 hrs prior to delivery
> Intrapartum fever
> Hx of infant with GBBS infection

Clinical manifestations (most common) of early-onset GBBS <7 days of life (late onset >7 days of life). Early onset accounts for 66% of all neonatal infection. Mortality rate 25–33%

> (1) Septicemia
> (2) Pneumonia
> (3) Meningitis

Late onset presents with meningitis in 85% (nosocomial/cross. colon)
Mortality 15–20% but survivors – 25–50% neurologic sequelae

CULTURE

Gold standard "Todd-Hewitt" Broth. Because cultures take 48 hrs, rapid GBBS antigen using coagulation, latex-particle agglutination and enzyme immunoassay. 1–2 hrs but has low sensitivity in lightly colonized patients, and could thus potentially fail to identify many patients who should receive prophylaxis

PREVENTION

> PCN G 5 million units IV then 2.5 million units IV every 4 hrs until delivery
> Ampicillin 2 g then 1 g every 4 hrs
> PCN Allergic – (clindamycin 900 mg every 8 hrs)
> (erythromycin 500 mg IV every 6 hrs until delivery)

GROUP B BETA STREPTOCOCCUS

Strategies to select from:

CDC –   Screening at 35–37 wks
Prophylaxis in pts found to be positive
Prophylaxis in pts with PROM or preterm labor prior to
term, with previous affected infant, or with GBBS
bacteriuria this pregnancy

ACOG –   Selective prophylaxis to all at risk, regardless of culture status
Risks include ROM ≥18 hrs, LBW, prematurity <37, chorioamnionitis,
IAI, previously affected infant, GBBS bacteriuria in pregnancy, temp
(intrapartum) >100.4 °F

AAP –   Universal screening at 26 wks
Prophylactic IV to selective patients in labor, depending on
risk factors and positive culture at 26 wks

GROUP B BETA STREPTOCOCCUS

AMERICAN COLLEGE OF OBSTETRICS AND GYNECOLOGY ALGORITHM FOR PREVENTION OF EARLY-ONSET GROUP B STREPTOCOCCAL DISEASE IN NEONATES, USING RISK FACTORS

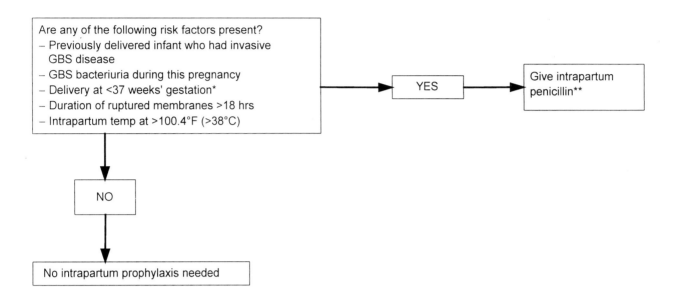

*If membrane ruptured at < 37 weeks' gestation, and the mother has not begun labor, collect group B streptococcal culture and either (a) administer antibiotics until cultures are completed and the results are negative or (b) begin antibiotics only when positive cultures are available

**Broader-spectrum antibiotics may be considered at the physician's discretion, based on clinical indications

RECOMMENDED REGIMENS FOR INTRAPARTUM ANTIMICROBIAL PROPHYLAXIS FOR PERINATAL GROUP B STREPTOCOCCAL DISEASE

RECOMMENDED: Penicillin G, 5 million units IV load, then 2.5 million units IV every 4 hrs until delivery

ALTERNATIVE: Ampicillin, 2 g IV load, then 1 g IV every 4 hrs until delivery

If penicillin-allergic:

RECOMMENDED: Clindamycin, 900 mg IV every 8 hrs until delivery

ALTERNATIVE: Erythromycin, 500 mg IV every 6 hrs until delivery

Note: If patient is receiving treatment for amnionitis with an antimicrobial agent active against group B streptococci (e.g. ampicillin, penicillin, clindamycin, or erythromycin) additional prophylactic antibiotics are not needed.

HEADACHES

FEATURES OF PRIMARY HEADACHES

	Migraine headache	*Tension-type headache*	*Cluster headache*
Aggravating or triggering factors	Alcohol, chocolate, other foods, altered sleep, change in weather, menstruation, physical activity	Emotional stress, rebound effect of overuse of analgesics (mostly unknown)	Alcohol (mostly unknown)
Ameliorating factors	Dark, quiet, rest	Hot or cold compresses	Physical activity
Associated symptoms			
Nausea	Usual	Slight and uncommon	Rare
Phonophobia	Usual	Slight and uncommon	Rare
Photophobia	Usual	Slight and uncommon	Rare
Nasal congestion/ rhinorrhea	Rare	Not present	Usual
Red/tearing eyes	Rare	Not present	Usual
Ptosis/miosis	Not present	Not present	Often
Aura	Occasional	Not present	Not present
Characteristics			
Type of pain	Throbbing	Steady ache	Boring
Location of pain	Unilateral	Bilateral	One orbit
Intensity of pain	Moderate-to-severe	Slight-to-moderate	Excruciating
Duration	4 hrs to 3 days	Hrs, wks, months	30 min to 3 hrs
Frequency	2/wk to 2/year	Daily to 2/year	Daily for wks or months
Family history	Usual	Occasional	Rare
Gender	F > M	F > M	M > F

HEADACHE QUESTIONNAIRE

Patient: _____   **Date:** _____

(Please answer all questions below – yes or no – with a check mark)

PAST HEADACHES
(Patient may have more than one type of headache or mixed headaches)

YES   NO

___ ___   1.   Do you have an idea of what may be causing your headache?
                (Whiplash, diabetes, high blood pressure, eye strain, etc.)
___ ___   2.   Did this same type of headache ever occur before?
___ ___   3.   Do you have more than one type of headache?
___ ___   4.   Is the headache pain so intense that sometimes it becomes unbearable?

TENSION HEADACHES
(Muscle contraction headache)
Head pain, tension, and muscle contractions of head, neck, or shoulders

___ ___   5.   Do your headaches occur during stressful tension or nervousness at home, at
                work, or during social occasions?
___ ___   6.   Do your neck, shoulder muscles or head junction feel tight and painful during
                the headache?
___ ___   7.   Is your headache pain dull and steady, like an intense constant pressure?
___ ___   8.   Does your headache feel like a tight band around the head?
___ ___   9.   Do you usually have one (1) or more headaches per week?
___ ___ 10.   Do your headaches occur during the day?
___ ___ 11.   Does mother, father, or any blood relative have similar headaches?
___ ___ 12.   Does exertion (lifting, running, straining, sex) affect your headache?
___ ___ 13.   Does nausea and/or vomiting occur before or during your headache?

MIGRAINE HEADACHES
(Common or Classic)
Usually women. Relieved by parenteral ergotamine confirms diagnosis

___ ___ 14.   Do you have any changes in vision (flashing lights, sensitivity to light, spots,
                blurred vision, etc.) before or during your headache?
___ ___ 15.   Does your headache usually start on one side of the head?
___ ___ 16.   Does your headache throb and pulsate or feel like it's pounding?
___ ___ 17.   Do your headaches usually occur during the night or upon awakening?
___ ___ 18.   Do your headaches usually occur during weekends and holidays?
___ ___ 19.   (Females only) Is your headache associated with your menstrual period?

CLUSTER HEADACHES
Usually men. 3 or more headaches per day for 4–8 wks

___ ___ 20.   Do you have watering of the eye on the affected side of the headache?
___ ___ 21.   Do alcoholic drinks cause or aggravate your headaches?

ORGANIC ORIGIN
Allergy, sinus infection, aneurysm, brain tumor, etc.

___ ___ 22.   Does chocolate, cheese, milk, nuts, Chinese food, or any other food cause
                or worsen your headaches?
___ ___ 23.   Do you have any hearing problems – noise, drainage or stuffiness in either ear?
___ ___ 24.   Have you noticed any paralysis, muscle weakness, numbness, swallowing
                problems or speech changes during your headaches?
___ ___ 25.   Do you have any facial pain, aching jaws, stuffiness or congested sinuses
                along with your headache?
___ ___ 26.   Has it been over eighteen (18) months since you last visited a dentist?

PREVIOUS TESTS & MEDICATIONS
___ ___ 27.   Have you had tests of headache? (X-ray, brain scan, injections, etc.)
___ ___ 28.   Have you used any previous headache medication? List all medications
                on the back of this form

HEADACHES

TREATMENT OPTIONS

Migraines

(1) Naproxen 500 mg p.o. daily
(2) Metoclopramide 10 mg p.o. daily
(3) Butorphanol NS 1 mg
(4) Sumatriptan (Imitrex) 6 mg SQ or 25 and 50 mg p.o. or 5, 10, and 20 mg NS
(5) Naratriptan hydrochloride (Amerge) 2.5 or 5 mg tablet p.o. q. 4 hrs (max. dose 2 tablets in 24 hrs)

Migraine prophylaxis

(1) Propranolol 20 mg p.o. t.i.d.
(2) Verapamil 80 mg p.o. t.i.d.
(3) Methylergonovine 0.2 mg p.o. t.i.d.
(4) Naproxen 250 mg p.o. t.i.d.
(5) Divalproex Na$^+$ 250 mg p.o. b.i.d.
(6) Amitriptyline 10–25 mg p.o. q.d.
(7) Methysergide 2 mg p.o. b.i.d.

Clusters

(1) Sumatriptan 6 mg SQ
(2) Ergotamine mg sublingual

Cluster prophylaxis

(1) Verapamil 80 mg p.o. t.i.d.
(2) Ergotamine tartrate with caffeine 100 mg – 1 mg p.o. b.i.d.

Chronic tension headache prophylaxis

(1) Amitriptyline 25 mg p.o. q.d.
(2) Divalproex Na$^+$ 250 mg p.o. b.i.d.
(3) Dihydroergotamine 0.5 mg t.i.d. IV

HEARTBURN IN PREGNANCY

SYMPTOMS

Indigestion, epigastric pain, dysphagia, water brash (hypersalivation), anorexia, nausea, vomiting, and rarely pulmonary symptoms

INCIDENCE

10–80%

COMPLICATIONS OF REFLUX

Esophagitis, bleeding, strictures (rare)

MECHANISMS (CAUSES)

TREATMENT STEPS

Hx:	Unable to lie down; forced to sleep upright
Exacerbate:	Fatty foods, caffeine, chocolate, natural mint, onions, garlic
Differential Dx:	PUD, gastritis, gallstones, constipation, pancreatitis, fatty liver of pregnancy, pre-eclampsia

Consider serum liver function tests, amylase, U/A. No endoscopy

(1) Avoid food/beverage 3 hrs prior to bed
(2) Avoid ETOH and smoking (decreased LES tone)
(3) Eat smaller and more frequent meals and avoid foods that exacerbate
(4) High protein and calcium-rich food may increase LES pressure and improve symptoms

Antacids
(½ pregnant women take antacids)

Liquids have greater gastric acid neutralizing capacity
Tablets (according to one study) = increased esophageal pH – improved relief reflux

Adverse reactions*:* Constipation, sodium bicarb – not alkalosis (avoid)

Gaviscon –	Increased doses associated with silicaceous nephrolithiasis, hypotonia, respiratory distress and cardiovascular problems in fetus

H_2 *blockers*:

(1)	*Cimetidine* –	Increased effect of theophyline, warfarin, dilantin, lidocaine. Used pre-op to prevent Mendelson's syndrome (gastric acid aspiration) Slow to cross placenta; and with antiandrogenic effects (800 b.i.d.; 400 q.i.d.)
(2)	*Zantac* –	More potent 150 b.i.d. Hemangioma of eyelid. Amniotic 4x – nl
(3)	*Pepcid* (AC)	10 mg b.i.d. Reflux Rx – 20 mg b.i.d.
(4)	*Axid*	(3x stronger than #1) 150 mg b.i.d. antiandrogenic/ inc abortion
(5)	*Carafate* –	1 g q.i.d. 1 degree PUD; coats ulcer crater – promotes healing As effective as H_2 blockers in relieving GER Costly. Has bioavailable aluminum @ with fetal death, abnormal skeletal growth and impaired hearing and memory in treated offspring of rats

Motility agents

(1) *Reglan* – Pre-op; increased gastric emptying; decreased emesis; increased lactation; 10–15 mg up to q.i.d. 30 min prior to each meal and at bedtime
Side-effects: Anxiety; insomnia; hallucinations; dystonic symptoms; Parkinson-like symptoms

(2) *Propulsid* – 10 mg q.i.d. 15 min prior to each meal and at bedtime.
Rx patients with nocturnal heartburn due to reflux.
*Releases endogenous acetylcholine and stimulates gas motility.
*Use only if potential benefits justify potential risks

Proton pump inhibitors

(1) *Prilosec* – helps heal erosive esophagitis

(2) *Prevacid* – recommended for severe erosive esophagitis
20 mg q.d. x 4–8 wks
Pre-op – ??

Further testing – symptoms persist; bleeding; esophageal strictures; Barrett's esophagus; ? Pre-cancer

Endoscopy

Demerol, Versed, Valium, Lidocaine 10% spray okay. Try to avoid barium studies with fluoroscopy

HEARTBURN IN PREGNANCY

MEDICATIONS TO RELIEVE HEARTBURN

Class of medication	FDA rating	Actions	Precautions
Antacids Aluminum hydroxide (ALternaGEL, Amphojel, Basaljel) Magnesium hydroxide with $Al(OH)_2$ (Aludrox, Maalox, Riopan) Calcium carbonate (Alka-Mints, Tums, Rolaids Calcium Rich/Sodium Free, Titralac) Magnesium trisilicate (with $Al(OH)_2$) (Gaviscon) Combination agents (Camalox, Tempo)	B1	Neutralizes gastric and esophageal acid May also contain simethicone, anti-gas agent (Di-Gel, Mylanta, Gelusil), alginic acid, or mucosal coating agent (Algicon)	
H_2 Blockers Cimetidine (Tagamet) Ranitidine (Zantac), Famotidine (Pepcid) Nizatidine (Axid)	B2 B1 C	Neutralizes gastric pH and decreases gastric volume	Cimetidine may be androgenic; nizatidine is embryotoxic in rabbits at high doses
Sucralfate	B1	Coats mucosa	Cost; possible aluminum absorption
Motility agents Metoclopramide (Reglan) Cisapride (Propulsid)	B C	Increases gastric emptying and LES pressure	CNS side-effects; cisapride embryotoxic in rats and rabbits at high doses
Proton pump inhibitors Omeprazole (Prilosec) Lansoprazole (Prevacid)	C	Suppresses gastric acid secretion	Embryotoxic in rats and rabbits at high doses

FDA pregnancy classifications

A	Well-controlled studies in women fail to show risk to the fetus
B1	Animal studies have not shown fetal risk, but there are no adequate studies in women
B2	Animal studies show some risk that has not been confirmed in controlled studies in women
C	Animal studies have shown adverse effects on the fetus, but there are no adequate controlled studies in women, or studies in women and animals are not available
D	Drugs that are associated with birth defects, but the potential benefits of the drug may outweigh possible risks
X	Drugs that may cause abnormalities in animals or humans. The potential risks clearly outweigh the drugs' potential benefits
LES	Lower esophageal sphincter

HELLP SYNDROME

ASSESS AND STABILIZE MATERNAL CONDITION

(1) If DIC is present, correct coagulopathy
(2) Provide antiseizure prophylaxis with magnesium sulfate
(3) Treat severe hypertension
(4) Transfer to tertiary care center if appropriate
(5) Perform computer tomography or ultrasound of the abdomen if subcapsular hematoma of the liver is suspected

EVALUATE FETAL WELL-BEING

EVALUATE FETAL LUNG MATURITY IF <35 WEEKS' GESTATION

(1) If mature, induce delivery
(2) If immature, give steroids, then allow for delivery
(3) Deliver if abnormal fetal assessment
(4) Deliver if progressive deterioration in maternal condition

HEMATURIA

DEFINITION

Presence of blood in urine (isolated hematuria) produced by bleeding in the urinary tract from urethra to renal pelvis

Total hematuria: occurs evenly throughout voiding (blood mixed fully with urine) suggests bleeding source proximal to bladder

Initial/completion hematuria: occurs at beginning or end of micturition, suggests bladder or urethral origin

CAUSES

(1)   Urinary calculi
(2)   Benign/malignant neoplasm
(3)   Infection
(4)   Tuberculosis
(5)   Trauma
(6)   Renal disease

DIAGNOSIS

History: Pattern of hematuria, symptomatology
Physical: Careful exam of external urethra
Labs:
(1)   Urinalysis – check for blood, pyuria, proteinuria
(2)   R/o coagulopathy – PT/PTT, platelets (CBC)
(3)   Microscopy – evaluate for presence of: RBCs, WBCs, casts (RBC, hyaline, fatty, WBC, epithelial cell, waxy)

RADIOLOGIC STUDIES

(1)   IVP, renal ultrasound – evaluate for hydronephrosis, renal/ureteral stones
(2)   CT, renal arteriography – sometimes necessary to disclose certain lesions (cysts, tumors)
(3)   Retrograde pyelography – when IVP not possible (Cr >1.5)

DIAGNOSTIC PROCEDURES

(1)   Cystoscopy – refer to Urology
(2)   Renal biopsy – refer to Nephrology

HEMATURIA

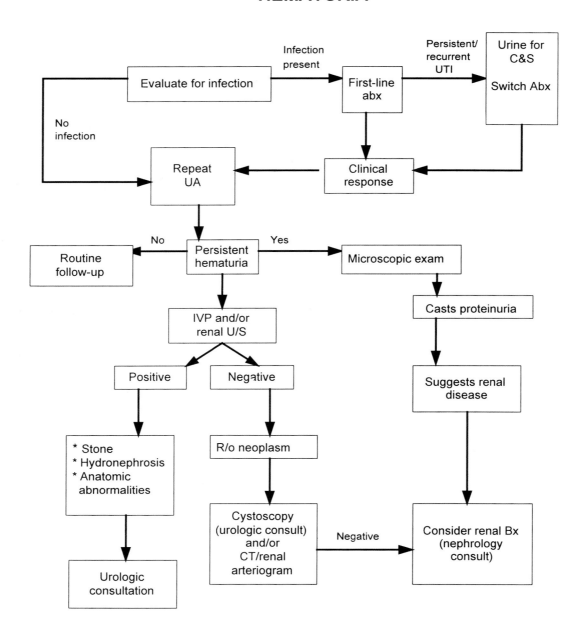

HEMORRHAGE (POSTPARTUM)

DEFINITION – Loss of >500 cc of blood during delivery

Underdiagnosed (~40% lose >500 cc/5% lose >1000 cc)
Early – within 24 hrs after delivery
Late – 24 hrs to 6 wks after delivery

ETIOLOGY: Uterine vs. extrauterine

Uterine

(1) **Atony** – over-distension (hydramnios, multiple gestation), temporal (rapid/prolonged labor), macrosomia, high parity, chorioamnionitis, tocolytics ($MgSO_4$, terbutaline), prolonged oxytocin administration, halothane anesthesia
(2) **Rupture** – previous uterine surgery, internal podalic version, breech extraction, obstructed labor (esp. high parity/multi-gestational), abnormal fetal presentation, mid-forceps rotations
(3) **Inversion** – complete vs incomplete

Extrauterine

(1) **Trauma** – (cervical/vaginal and/or rectal lacerations), forceps, macrosomia, precipitous labor, episiotomy
(2) **Hematoma** – vulvar (subacute volume loss/pain), vaginal (severe rectal pressure), retroperitoneal (least common, but most dangerous/no warning signs)
(3) **Retained placental fragments** – accreta, increta, percreta, abnormalities (succenturiate lobe)
(4) **Coagulopathy** – obstetric conditions (abruption, amniotic fluid embolism, pre-eclampsia, retained dead fetus). Medical conditions (acquired/inherited coag disorders, autoimmune thrombocytopenia, anti-coagulant use)

MANAGEMENT

Determine cause
(1) Vigorous fundal massage
(2) Bimanual uterine compression
(3) Suspect lower genital tract lacs
(4) Inspect placenta
(5) Inspect uterus (rupture/retained placenta?)
(6) Think coagulopathy
(7) Inspect for uterine inversion

Medical management

(1) Pitocin – 20 U in 1000 cc LR or NS as IV infusion
(2) Methylergo novine (Methergine) – 0.2 mg IM
(3) 15-Methyl PGF (Hemabate) – 0.25 mg IM/intramyometrial q. 15–60 min p.r.n.

Volume replacement

(1) Large bore IV line
(2) Foley catheter
(3) Infusion of LR or NS at 3 cc/cc estimated blood loss (maintain UOP ≥30 cc/hr)

(4) Blood transfusion – uncrossmatched in emergency
(5) FFP, platelets, cryoprecipitate as indicated

Surgical management

(1) Ligation – uterine, utero-ovarian, infundipulopelvic and/or hypogastric vessels
(2) Hysterectomy (consider parity, future child-bearing, extent of hemorrhage)
  – Failure to respond to medical/conservative surgical management
  – Placenta accreta
  – Uterine rupture

DELAYED POSTPARTUM HEMORRHAGE – (>24 hrs postpartum)

Etiology

Subinvolution of placental site, retained POC, endometritis

Management

Pitocin, Methergine, Hemabate, antibiotics (endometritis), r/o coagulopathy, curettage (if necessary), may attempt angiographic embolization prior to surgery/hysterectomy

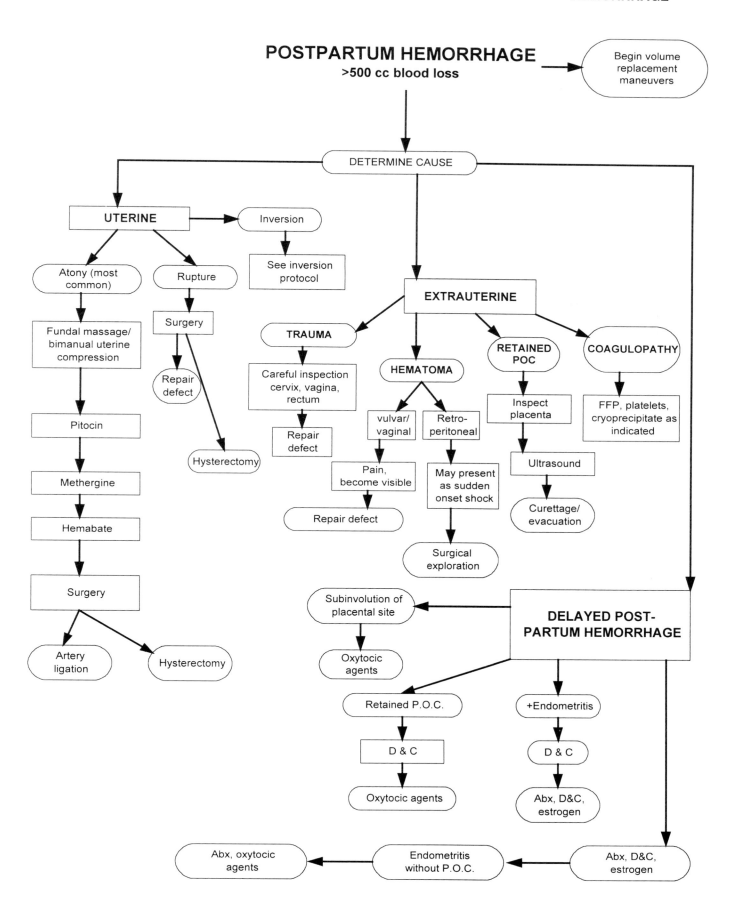

HEPATITIS IN PREGNANCY

HEPATITIS B

DNA virus (Dane particle)
3 principal antigens (HbsAg, HbcAg, HbeAg)
Acute infection 1–2/1000 pregnancies
Chronic infection 5–15/1000 pregnancies
Transmitted parenterally or by sexual contact
Risk factors
    – History of IV drug abuse
    – History of sexually transmitted disease
    – Multiple sexual partners
    – Health care/public safety career
    – Household Hepatitis B carrier
    – Work/treatment in hemodialysis
    – Bleeding disorder (Recipient of blood products)
Acute infection mortality = 1% (85–90% complete resolution)
Chronic infection in 10–15% (15–30% active viral DNA replication)
Perinatal transmission 10–20% of HepBsAg seropositive
       (90% if mother HbsAg and HbeAg positive)

CLINICAL MANIFESTATION

Symptoms: malaise, fatigue, anorexia, nausea, RUQ/epigastric pain
Signs: jaundice, upper abdominal tenderness, hepatomegaly, dark urine, alcoholic stool (fulminant hepatitis = coagulopathy, encephalopathy)

DIAGNOSIS

Laboratory tests – marked increase ALT, AST, serum bilirubin (severe hepatitis = coagulation abnormalities, hyperammonemia)
Liver biopsy – rarely indicated

Specific serology

Hepatitis virus	Acute	Chronic
A	HepA Ig M Ab	None
B	H Bs Ag H Be Ag (high infectivity) H Bc Ag IgM Ab	H Bs Ag
C	Hep C Ab	Persistent hepatic dysfunction
D	Hep D Ag Hep D IgM Ab	Hep D Ag Hep D IgG Ab

MANAGEMENT

Supportive

Hospitalization for severe cases (encephalopathy, coagulopathy, etc)
Mild to moderate illness may be managed as out-patient
  – reduce activity
  – avoid upper abdominal trauma
  – maintain nutrition/hydration
  – avoid intimate contact with household or sexual partners until immunoprophylaxis initiated

Specific immunotherapy

Hepatitis A *Vaccine* – investigative trials

Immunoglobulin – pre/post exposure prophylaxis for travel to endemic areas (safe in pregnancy)

Hepatitis B – cannot alter natural course once patient is clinically ill

Vaccination – indicated for women with risk factors
  – susceptible pregnant patients targeted for vaccine

Immunoglobulin – exposure to Hep B prior to vaccination exposure via sexual contact – single dose HBIG within 14 days exposure via injury (needle stick, etc) – immediate dose followed by second dose 1 month later

Passive/active immunization especially important in pregnant pts (reduces perinatal transmission 85–95%)

Neonatal immunoprophylaxis

Vaccination recommended for all newborns (CDC)
  1st vaccination = birth to 12 hrs
  2nd vaccination = 1 month
  3rd vaccination = 6 months

Immunoglobulin – indicated for newborns of HbsAg positive or unknown status mother
  – HBIG 0.5 ml IM = birth to 12 hrs
  (Hep B screening recommended for all pregnant women)

Hepatitis C/D No antiviral agents available
  (Measures to prevent Hep B effective in preventing Hep D)

HEPATITIS TYPES AND CHARACTERISTICS

Hepatitis A

1/3 of hepatitis in USA
RNA virus
Fecal–oral
Dxn: IgM increased ALT AST Bilirubin
Rx: Supportive care
  Within 2 wks of exp, give **immunoglobulin + Hep A vaccine** to sexual and household contacts (vaccine safe in pregnancy)
  Hepatitis A vaccine is **contraindicated** with other **live** vaccines
Perinatal transmission does not occur
Chronic carrier state does not exist

Hepatitis B

40–45% of hepatitis in USA
DNA virus (Dane particle = intact virus)
Parental, sexual contact, or perinatal

Dxn: Detection of Hep B surface antigen + IgM to core antigen
HbeAg indicates exceptionally increased virus load – very infectious

Rx: HBIG stat then Hep B vaccine for contacts and newborns. Newborns need only vaccine if mom neg

Perinatal transmission (10–20% if + HbsAg; 90% if +HbeAg and HbsAg)

Hepatitis C

10–20 % of cases in USA
RNA virus
Post-transfusion (90%)

Dxn: +Anti-C antibody
Screen with EIA (enzyme immunoassay). Follow +EIA with RIBA (recombinant immunoblot assay)

Rxn: None. **No vaccine for hepatitis C**

Perinatal transmission 10–44%

Hepatitis non-A, non-B

Occurs in two forms:
(1) Parentally transmitted Hepatitis C
(2) Enterically transmitted Hepatitis E

Hepatitis D

Coinfection with Hep B
Coinfection and/or superinfection with Hepatitis D
Coinfection with acute Hep B + D (usu self-limited and rarely leads to chronic liver dis.)
Superinfection – develops when acute Hep D develops in a patient who is a chronic Hep B carrier

Hepatitis E

Rare in USA
RNA virus
Fecal–oral

Dxn: Electron microscopy, fluorescent antibody blocking assay, and Western blot assay

Rx: Same as Hep A

No perinatal transmission or chronic carrier state

Hepatitis G

Associated with chronic viremia lasting at least 10 years. Detected in 15% of patients with chronic B or C; (percutaneous)

HERPES

DIAGNOSIS

Classical signs and symptoms

    (1)   Painful or pruritic vesicles clustered on the labia and/or buttocks

Other common signs and symptoms

    (2)   Dysuria
    (3)   Tender inguinal lymph nodes
    (4)   Cervical ulcerations

Tzanck Smear: rapid and inexpensive test

    (1)   Scrape opened vesicle on slide
    (2)   Giemsa, Sedi, or Wright's stain is applied
    (3)   Characteristic cytopathology:
            (a)   Multinucleated giant cells
            (b)   Atypical Keratinocytes
            (c)   "Ground glass" cytoplasm

Viral HSVII culture: obtain when vesicle is wet. 90% (Only 25–30% recovery with crusted lesions)

    *Also test for syphilis, GC/*Chlamydia*, bacterial vaginosis, and *Trichomonas*

Educate patient

    (1)   Warn about spread
    (2)   Advise use of condoms
    (3)   Recurrences
    (4)   Advise about danger of perinatal transmission, asymptomatic shedding especially increased with prolonged first degree outbreak and frequent symptomatic recurrences

PRESCRIPTIONS

    (1)   Acyclovir 200 mg, 5x per day for 10 days
            Recurrences: acyclovir 400 mg p.o. 3x day for 7–10 days
            Prevention/control: acyclovir 200 mg 5x day for 5 days
            Suppressive (>12 outbreaks/year); acyclovir 400 mg p.o. twice daily

    (2)   Valacyclovir 1 g twice daily x10 days
            Recurrences: 500 mg twice daily x5 days

    (3)   Famcyclovir
            Recurrences: 125 mg twice daily x5 days

PREGNANCY

    (1)   Culture active lesions to confirm diagnosis
    (2)   Vaginal delivery if no lesions
    (3)   C/S if prodromal symptoms or visible HSV lesions
    (4)   Suppressive Rx >36 wks – acyclovir 400 mg 3x day

HIRSUTISM

DEFINITION

Excessive hair involving areas that follow a male pattern of hair distribution

EVALUATION

Define the source of abnormal androgen production, and specifically suppress the increased production

DIFFERENTIAL DIAGNOSIS

(6 disorders)

(1) Drug induced – i.e. exogenous testosterone, Danazol
(2) Intersex conditions – i.e. ambiguous genitalia
(3) Ovary – i.e. PCO syndrome, stromal hyperthecosis, ovarian tumors
(4) Adrenal – i.e. adrenal tumors, Cushing syndrome, congenital adrenal hyperplasia
(5) Peripheral – i.e. idiopathic
(6) Pregnancy – i.e. luteoma, hyperreactio luteinalis

CLINICAL MARKERS

(1) Testosterone – an ovarian marker
(2) DHEAS – an adrenal marker
(3) 3-alpha androstenediol glucuronide – a peripheral marker (is not part of a routine workup – Speroff page 488)

The most common cause of hirsutism in women is anovulation and excessive androgen production by the ovaries
Adrenal causes are the least common

DIAGNOSTIC WORKUP

(1) Initial lab evaluation of hirsutism – serum total testosterone, DHEAS, and 17-OHP (17-hydroxyprogesterone). Evaluation for anovulation – prolactin, and thyroid function
(2) History and physical

LABORATORY FINDINGS

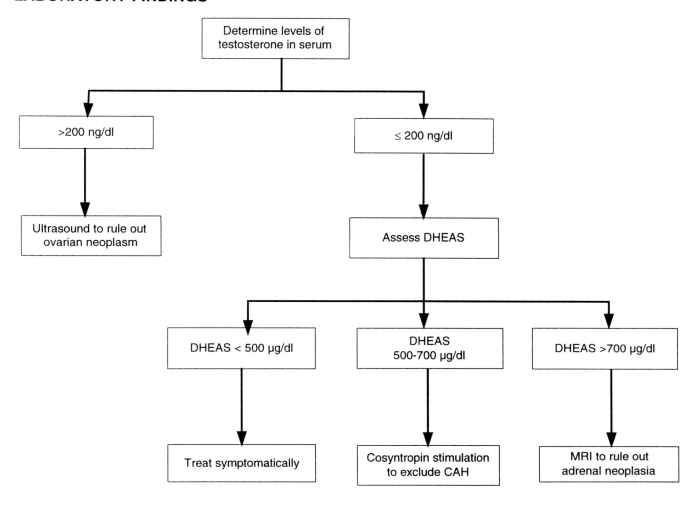

TREATMENT

Treatment of hirsutism according to source of androgen excess

Androgen	Treatment
↑ Testosterone	Oral contraceptives
↑ DHEA-S (<5 µg/ml)	Oral contraceptives
↑ DHEA-S (>5 µg/ml)	Dexamethasone
↑ Testosterone. ↑ DHEA-S (7 µg/ml)	Oral contraceptives + dexamethasone
↑ 3α-diol G, normal T, normal DHEA-S	Spironolactone*

From Lobo RA. Androgen excess. In Mishell DR Jr, Davajan V, Lobo RA. eds. *Infertility, Contraception and Reproductive Endocrinology*, 3rd edn. Cambridge, Mass: Blackwell Scientific Publications, 1991
*Spironolactone may also be substituted for any of the above regimens if no improvement is noted after 3–4 months of treatment

Agents available to inhibit various sources of androgen production

Ovarian
>   Oral contraceptives
>   Progestins including depo-medroxyprogesterone acetate
>   Gonadotropin releasing hormone agonist
>   Antiandrogenism (cyproterone acetate, spironolactone)
>   Ketoconazole
>   Corticosteroids

Adrenal
>   Corticosteroids
>   Oral contraceptives
>   Spironolactone
>   Ketoconazole

Peripheral
>   Cyproterone acetate
>   Spironolactone
>   Progesterone (topical)
>   Oral contraceptives
> 5α-Reductase inhibitors

Modified from Lobo RA. Androgen excess. In Mishell DR Jr, Davajan V, Lobo RA. eds. *Infertility, Contraception and Reproductive Endocrinology*, 3rd edn. Cambridge, Mass: Blackwell Scientific Publications, 1991

HIRSUTISM PROTOCOL

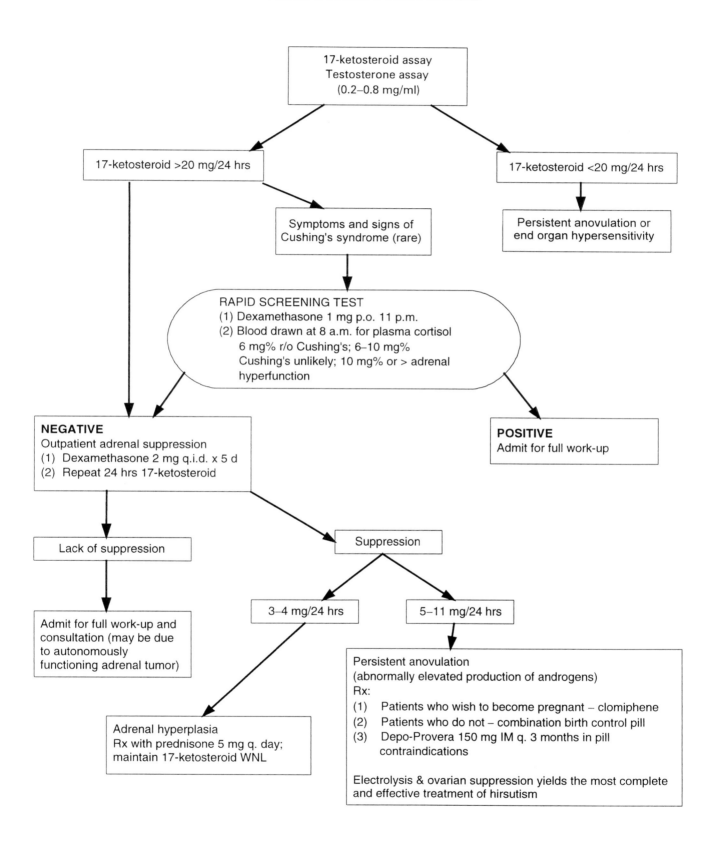

17-ketosteroid assay
Testosterone assay
(0.2–0.8 mg/ml)

17-ketosteroid >20 mg/24 hrs

17-ketosteroid <20 mg/24 hrs

Symptoms and signs of
Cushing's syndrome (rare)

Persistent anovulation or
end organ hypersensitivity

RAPID SCREENING TEST
(1) Dexamethasone 1 mg p.o. 11 p.m.
(2) Blood drawn at 8 a.m. for plasma cortisol
6 mg% r/o Cushing's; 6–10 mg%
Cushing's unlikely; 10 mg% or > adrenal
hyperfunction

NEGATIVE
Outpatient adrenal suppression
(1) Dexamethasone 2 mg q.i.d. x 5 d
(2) Repeat 24 hrs 17-ketosteroid

POSITIVE
Admit for full work-up

Lack of suppression

Suppression

Admit for full work-up and
consultation (may be due
to autonomously
functioning adrenal tumor)

3–4 mg/24 hrs

5–11 mg/24 hrs

Persistent anovulation
(abnormally elevated production of androgens)
Rx:
(1) Patients who wish to become pregnant – clomiphene
(2) Patients who do not – combination birth control pill
(3) Depo-Provera 150 mg IM q. 3 months in pill
     contraindications

Electrolysis & ovarian suppression yields the most complete
and effective treatment of hirsutism

Adrenal hyperplasia
Rx with prednisone 5 mg q. day;
maintain 17-ketosteroid WNL

HYPEREMESIS GRAVIDARUM

Consists of nausea and vomiting to the extent of weight loss, dehydration, electrolyte imbalance, acid–base disturbance and – in severe cases – renal and hepatic injury

LABORATORY TESTS & NURSING REQUIREMENT

(1) Serum electrolytes (start) on admission
(2) CBC, LFTs, amylase and lipase, U/A, thyroid function (optional)
(3) Urinary ketones (dipstick) on every void while NPO
(4) Daily weight
(5) Accurate intake/output

INTRAVENOUS HYDRATION

(1) D5NS 250 cc/hr x4 hrs (start on admission), then 150 cc/hr (may be given more if severely dehydrated)
(2) Add KCl (20–40 mEq) to the second and subsequent liters if the serum K^+ is in the low normal range or below
(3) Add MVT to 1 l/day (optional)
     Add folic acid 1 mg (optional)
     Add pyridoxine (Vit B_6) 25 mg/l (optional)

DIET

(1) Day of admission (Day #1):   NPO
(2) Day #2:   Start in morning if no nausea/vomiting
              Clear liquids (no hot or cold liquids; no ice or straws); no coffee
              Cola of choice (at room temperature)
              Saltine crackers
(3) Day #3:   Start in morning if no nausea/vomiting
              Low-fat/bland/dry food; small portions
              Divide calories into three meals plus three snacks

DRUG THERAPY

(1) **Droperidol**
     Solution: 25 mg in 500 cc D5W (or NS) (0.05 mg/ml)
     Start at 1 mg (20 ml) per hour (use infusion pump)
     Give 1–2.5 mg bolus dose over 30 min if vomiting is present
     If no vomiting, start without bolus dose

     Dose adjustment: 0.25 mg (5 ml) increments every 4 hrs
     An informed consent is obtained from the pt before the Droperidol is started
     The consent reviews the potential material toxicities and in general terms, the known etiologies of birth defects

(2) **Diphenhydramine** (Benadryl)
     50 mg IV over 30 min every 6 hrs (not p.r.n.)
     First dose immediately prior to starting Droperidol
     Give extra dose at anytime if required (if pt experiences extra pyramidal symptoms)
     Use (1) and (2) together

(3) **Benztropine**
   Use if pt unresponsive to diphenhydramine 1 mg IV (or IM) initially, then 10 mg/IM q. 12 hr
   If not responsive to (2)

(4) **Metoclopramide** (Reglan)
   10 mg p.o. ½ hr before meals and at bedtime (4x daily)

(5) **Hydroxyzine** (Atarax)
   50 mg p.o. ½ hr before meals and at bedtime
   Use (4) and (5) together

(6) **Zofran**
   32 mg IV over 15 min then 0.15 mg/kg IV every 4–8 hrs x3 doses

(7) **Cocktail** (GI Mixture)
   Combination of Bentyl 15 cc, lidocaine 15 cc, and Mylanta 3 oz *or* combination of Donnatal 4 oz
      and Mylanta 8 oz.

(8) **Methylprednisolone** – 48 mg daily x3 days; then taper for 12 days

If the patient tolerates her first solid food meals, the Droperidol is discontinued approximately 2 hrs before the next meal. Then Reglan and Atarax are started about 30 min before the next meal

DOSE-RELATED TOXICITY

Common (~15%):   akathisia (mild) (restlessness/hyperactivity/anxiety)

Uncommon (<1%):   dystonia
                  dizziness
                  laryngospasm
                  oculogyria

Reported in literature: hypotension
                          tachycardia
                          chills
                          shivering
                          bronchospasm
                          hallucinations

HYPERTENSION IN PREGNANCY

Hypertensive disease complicates 6–8% of all pregnancies in the United States and is one of the major causes of maternal death

The Committee on Terminology of the American College of Obstetricians and Gynecologists list the following classifications:

    (1)   Pre-eclampsia
        (a)   Mild
        (b)   Severe
        (c)   Eclampsia
    (2)   Chronic hypertension
    (3)   Chronic hypertension with superimposed pre-eclampsia/eclampsia
    (4)   Transient or gestational hypertension

Hypertension is defined as a sustained blood pressure increase to levels of 140 mmHg systolic or 90 mmHg diastolic

Pregnancy-induced hypertension has its onset after 20 weeks of gestation and chronic hypertension is defined as hypertension developing before 20 weeks of gestation

The etiology of pregnancy-induced hypertension is unknown. However, it is well established that the disease process occurs most often in women who are pregnant for the first time, women with multiple gestation, and women with certain vascular disorders such as those seen with insulin-dependent diabetes, lupus erythematosus, renal disease and chronic hypertension. The major pathophysiologic derangement is vasospasm

Severe pre-eclampsia is diagnosed when one or more of the following situations exist:
    (1)   Blood pressure >160–180 mmHg systolic or >110 mmHg diastolic
    (2)   Proteinuria >5 g/24 hr (normal <300 mg/24 hr)
    (3)   Elevated serum creatinine
    (4)   Grand mal seizures (eclampsia)
    (5)   Pulmonary edema
    (6)   Oliguria <500 ml/24hr
    (7)   Microangiopathic hemolysis
    (8)   Thrombocytopenia
    (9)   Hepatocellular dysfunction (elevated alanine aminotransferase, aspartase)
    (10)   Intrauterine growth restriction or oligohydramnios
    (11)   Symptoms suggesting significant end-organ involvement:
        (a)   Headache
        (b)   Visual disturbances
        (c)   Epigastric or right upper quadrant pain

CLINICAL MANAGEMENT

Delivery is always an appropriate option in the term patient with hypertension. However, in the patient with an unfavorable cervix who exhibits only mild blood pressure elevations, minimal proteinuria, and no evidence of either maternal end-organ involvement or fetal compromise, it may be appropriate to delay delivery in an effort to obtain a more favorable cervix before induction

Delivery should be considered in women who have signs and symptoms of severe pre-eclampsia at 32–34 weeks of gestation

In some cases, the condition of a woman who initially manifests signs and symptoms of severe pre-eclampsia will improve after observation and treatment with magnesium sulfate and various antihypertensive agents. In such women, continued observation is reasonable and appropriate at less than 32 weeks of gestation. If severe pre-eclampsia recurs or does not respond to initial observation and therapy, delivery should be instituted

Some of the manifestations of severe pre-eclampsia, such as maternal oliguria, renal failure and HELLP syndrome, require expedient delivery regardless of gestational age

For the preterm patient with mild pre-eclampsia, conservative management is generally indicated. It is essential to closely monitor blood pressure and proteinuria and evaluate renal and hepatic function and platelet count. Serial sonography for fetal growth and antepartum assessment of fetal well-being are also important. For stable patients with mild pre-eclampsia who have had a thorough initial evaluation, either inpatient or outpatient management may be appropriate

When delivery is indicated, parenteral magnesium sulfate generally is administered to prevent seizures. Given as intravenous loading bolus followed by a continuous infusion. The therapeutic range for magnesium is 4–8 mg/dl. Infusion should be discontinued and a serum magnesium level should be obtained in any patient with loss of deep tendon reflexes, a respiration rate of less than 12/min and a decreased urinary output to below 25 ml/hr. When symptomatic magnesium overdose is suspected, it can be reversed by the intravenous administration of calcium gluconate

When blood pressure exceeds 110 mmHg diastolic or 180 mmHg systolic, consideration should be given to lowering the blood pressure

Hydralazine is widely used, given intravenously 5 mg. Intravenous Labetalol is an acceptable substitute. The maximum effect of a single dose occurs within 5 minutes

Vaginal delivery is generally preferable to Cesarean delivery even in patients with manifestation of severe disease

Women undergoing Cesarean delivery may receive either general or conduction anesthesia, depending on the circumstances, expertise and skills of the anesthesiologist, and, most importantly the woman's desire after informed consent

HYPERTHYROIDISM

Graves disease: 85% cases

Nodular goiter and *Hashimoto's thyroiditis* are occasionally responsible

R/o *hydatidiform mole* – may produce symptoms and lab tests consistent with thyrotoxicosis

Hyperemesis gravidarum – may present with hyperthyroid values that normalize after correction of dehydration

SYMPTOMS

Nervousness, palpitations, heat intolerance, goiter, weight loss, and inability to gain weight. In pregnancy, most commonly – persistent tachycardia and lack of weight gain

DIAGNOSIS

Increased FT-4 or free thyroxine index

Decreased TSH

Increased TSH R Ab (thyroid stimulating hormone receptor antibody) – a marker for Graves disease, can be used to determine who is at risk of having an infant with fetal or neonatal hyperthyroidism

TREATMENT

Tapazole 10–20 mg p.o. b.i.d. (increase to 60 mg if severe)

PTU (propylthiouracil) 100–150 mg p.o. t.i.d. (inc to 600 mg p.r.n.)

Add propranolol (10–40 mg p.o. q. 6–8 hrs) p.r.n.

F/u q. 2–3 wks with free thyroxine index

When FT-4 index improves, decrease antithyroid drug to ½ dose then until Tapazole is 15 mg or PTU is 50 mg daily. Goal is to keep FT-4 index in upper 1/3 normal until 30–34 weeks' gestation then if euthyroid, then d/c until delivery. Double last total daily amount p.r.n.

HYPOTHYROIDISM

SYMPTOMS

Tiredness, lethargy, constipation, cold intolerance, menorrhagia and infertility

More advanced symptoms

Drowsiness, decrease in intellect and motor activity, hair loss, brittle nails, husky voice, weight gain, stiffness and tingling of the fingers, dry skin

DIAGNOSIS

Decreased serum thyroxine; increased TSH

PREGNANCY

Increase in spontaneous abortions; increase PIH

TREATMENT

L-thyroxine   (1.6–2 mg/kg of ideal body weight)
(0.075–0.15 mg/d)

If patient is taking thyroid replacement at time of initial visit for pregnancy, check TSH. 50% of pregnant patients will need an increase in dosage

If TSH is elevated, increase L-thyroxine by 50 mg; repeat TSH in 4–6 wks

If TSH is normal, repeat TSH at 22–28 wks gestation

After delivery, return to pre-pregnancy L-thyroxine dose

Start newly diagnosed hypothyroid patients with full replacement dose

Repeat TSH every 4 wks and adjust the amount of L-thyroxine to keep the serum TSH within normal limits

IMMUNIZATIONS

GENERAL PRINCIPLES

Immunologic therapy, 4 types
- (1) *Inactivated vaccines* – Hepatitis B, Influenza, *Pneumococcus*
- (2) *Live-attenuated vaccines* – measles, mumps, rubella, polio
- (3) *Toxoids* – tetanus, diphtheria
- (4) *Immunoglobulins* – Hepatitis B, rabies, tetanus, varicella, Hepatitis A, measles

Childhood immunizations – most women immune to: measles, mumps, rubella, tetanus, diphtheria, polio by child-bearing age

Vaccinate according to age group and risk factors

Age 13–18

Tetanus–diphtheria booster (age 14–16 x1)

At-risk groups:
- (1) Child-bearing age and no evidence of immunity – MMR
- (2) Blood products, household/sexual contacts of Hep B carriers, multiple sexual partners in past 6 months – Hep B vaccine

Age 19–65

Tetanus–diphtheria booster (every 10 yrs)
Influenza vaccine (every year starting at age 55)

At-risk groups:
- (1) Child-bearing age and no evidence of immunity – MMR
- (2) IV drug users; blood products recipients; healthcare workers; household/sexual contacts of Hep B carriers; multiple sexual partners in past 6 months – Hep B vaccine
- (3) Chronic cardiopulmonary disease; metabolic diseases; diabetes, hemoglobinopathies, immunosuppression, renal dysfunction – influenza vaccine annually
- (4) Conditions prone to pneumococcal infection (i.e. immunosuppression) chronic cardiopulmonary disease, sickle cell disease, renal disease, s/p splenectomy, diabetes, alcoholism, cirrhosis – Pneumovax

Age 65+

Tetanus–diphtheria booster (every 10 yrs)
Influenza vaccine (annually)
Pneumovax (once)

At-risk groups:
- (1) Exposure to blood products; household/sexual contacts with chronic Hep B carriers – Hep B vaccine

IMMUNIZATIONS IN PREGNANCY

Theoretical concern of congenital infection by live vaccines during pregnancy (no reported cases)

Must weigh several factors: risk of exposure, maternal risk, fetal risk, risk from vaccine/toxoid

Rule of thumb: No live vaccines unless:
(1)   Susceptibility/exposure probable, and
(2)   Disease threat to woman/fetus – vaccine risk

Only routinely administered immunizations during pregnancy:
(1)   Tetanus–diphtheria toxoids
(2)   At-risk group for Hep B virus (see above)

MMR: 3 months before pregnancy or immediate postpartum

Polio/yellow fever vaccine – when traveling to endemic area

Immune globulins:
(1)   After exposure to: measles, Hep A, B, tetanus, chicken pox or rabies
(2)   VZIG for newborns of mother who develop chickenpox 5 days before, until 2 days after delivery
(3)   All women without a history of chicken pox should be passively immunized with VZIG within 96 hours of an exposure to chicken pox

IMMUNIZATIONS

INDICATIONS FOR VACCINES AND IMMUNE SERUM GLOBULINS DURING PREGNANCY

Immunizing agent	Indications
Vaccines	
Live virus	
Poliomyelitis (Sabin)	Immediate protection against poliomyelitis for previously unimmunized individuals
Yellow fever	Travel to endemic areas
Measles	Contraindicated
Mumps	Contraindicated
Rubella	Contraindicated
Live bacteria	
Tularemia	Rabbit handlers, laboratory workers
Bacille Calmette-Guérin	Not recommended
Killed virus	
Hepatitis B	Pre- and postexposure prophylaxis for individuals at high-risk
Influenza	Chronic cardiopulmonary or renal disease; diabetes mellitus
Poliomyelitis (Salk)	Travel to epidemic areas; laboratory workers
Rabies	Exposure to potentially rabid animals
Killed bacteria	
Cholera	Entry requirement for some countries
Meningococcus	Epidemic meningococcal–non-B disease
Plaque	Laboratory workers; travel to areas with human disease
Pneumococcus	Cardiopulmonary disease, splenectomy, alcoholism, Hodgkin's
Typhoid	Household contact with chronic carrier; travel to endemic areas
Pertussis	Not recommended
Toxoids	
Anthrax	Laboratory workers; handlers of furs and animal hides
Tetanus–diphtheria	Primary immunization; booster
Immune globulins	
Pooled human	
Hepatitis A	Pre- and postexposure prophylaxis
Measles	Postexposure prophylaxis
Hyperimmune	
Hepatitis B	Postexposure prophylaxis
Rabies	Postexposure prophylaxis
Tetanus	Postexposure prophylaxis
Varicella zoster	Postexposure prophylaxis
Horse serum	
Botulism	Treatment of infection
Diphtheria	Treatment of infection

IMMUNIZATIONS

IMMUNIZATIONS FOR CHILDREN

Although we do not give immunizations to pediatric patients, we are often asked by mothers about the times when children are due for their immunizations. This list should help answer those questions

Hepatitis B

1 month (Hep B-1)
2 months (Hep B-2)
12–15 months (Hep B-3)
11–12 years (Hep B*)   (*For those who have not completed the full series of three doses*)

DTaPor DTP

2 months
4 months
6 months
15–18 months
4–6 years
11–16 years Td (*Tetanus booster*)

H. influenzae type B

2 months
4 months
6 months
12–15 months

Polio

2 months
4 months
15 months
4–6 years

Measles, mumps, rubella

12–15 months
4–6 years or 11–12 years

Varicella

15 months
11–12 years

INCONTINENCE

GENERAL PRINCIPLES

(1) Offer less invasive approaches first (reserve surgery for failed conservative measures)
(2) Avoid excess fluid intake (limit ~2 l/day)
(3) Decrease caffeine consumption
(4) Assess necessity of diuretic therapy
(5) Void at regular intervals

PELVIC MUSCLE EXERCISES

Useful in stress or urge incontinence (40–75%)

Contraction of the pubococcygeus for 10 seconds for 10–20 repetitions

Instruct to achieve total of 100 contractions/day

At least 6 wks needed to see improvement

Teach patients correct method during pelvic exam or instruct to attempt to interrupt urine stream

MEDICATIONS

(1) *Urge incontinence:* oxybutynin HCl (Ditropan) 5 mg p.o. b.i.d.–t.i.d. or propantheline bromide (Pro-Banthine) 15 mg p.o. t.i.d. or tolterodine tartrate (Detrol) 2 mg p.o. b.i.d.
(2) *Mixed stress incontinence/detrusor instability:* imipramine (Tofranil) 50–150 mg p.o. q. d
(3) *Mild/moderate stress incontinence:* phenylpropanolamine (Propagest) 75–150 mg p.o. q. d
(4) *Estrogen deficiency:* estrogen vaginal cream ½–1 applicatorful, biw–tiw x6–12 wks

SURGERY

Success inversely proportional to number of procedures

Procedures to restore anatomic support proximal urethra/cystocele:

(1) Anterior colporrhaphy/Kelly plication (cure rate 40–70%)
(2) Abdominal retropubic urethropexy (Marshall–Marchetti–Krantz, Burch procedure)
    Cure rate: primary incontinence: 70–90%
                 recurrent incontinence: 40–70%
(3) Needle suspension/sling procedures (Stamey, Raz, Pereyra, suburethral sling)
    After failure of above techniques, refer to urogynecology specialist
    Cure rate: 70–95%

Procedures to compensate for intrinsic sphincter deficiency (ISD)

(1) Periurethral collagen injection
    Cure rate: well-supported urethra = 70–90%
                 urethral hypermobility = 20–50%*
    *Often requires combination procedure (Kelly plication, MMK, Burch)
(2) Artificial urethral sphincter

INCONTINENCE

DIAGNOSIS OF URINARY INCONTINENCE

Stress incontinence (SUI)

Involuntary loss of urine during physical activity due to loss of anatomic support of the urethra, bladder or urethrovesical junction or due to intrinsic sphincter deficiency

Urge incontinence

Involuntary loss of urine associated with an abrupt and strong desire to void due to detrusor instability

Overflow incontinence

Involuntary loss of urine associated with a large post-void residual due to detrusor underactivity

Functional incontinence

Involuntary loss of urine due to physical limitations hindering patient's ability to reach bathroom facilities (e.g. arthritis, mobility restrictions)

Extraurethral incontinence

Involuntary loss of urine due to anatomic bypass of normal continence mechanisms (e.g. vesicovaginal fistula, ectopic ureter, urethral diverticulum)

Diagnosis

(1)   *History:* medical/surgical, obstetric, medications
(2)   *Physical:*
    (a)   *Neurologic* (sphincter tone, motor/sensory exam)
    (b)   *Pelvic* – assess for estrogen deficiency, loss of pelvic support, cystocele/rectocele
(3)   *Labs:* urine analysis/culture
(4)   *Office cystometrics*
    (a)   Have patient empty bladder
    (b)   *Q-Tip test:* with patient in lithotomy position, aseptically introduce cotton-tip applicator (lubricated) through urethra. Ask patient to cough. If Q-tip deviates >45 degrees = urethral hypermobility. Some physicians suggest this test is better if done with patient in standing position
    (c)   *Post-void residual:* remove cotton-tip applicator; insert red rubber catheter, measure residual urine (send portion for culture). Greater than 100 cc, consider overflow incontinence
    (d)   *Cystometry:* attach 60 ml Toomey syringe to catheter (plunger removed). Add sterile saline/water in 50 ml increments. Record volume at 1st urge and sensation of inability to remain continent

        OUTCOMES
        (i)   Rise in fluid level associated with urgency = detrusor instability
        (ii)   Bladder capacity <300 cc, consider bladder spasm
        (iii)   Bladder capacity >600 cc, consider neurogenic bladder
        (iv)   Normal bladder capacity – perform stress tests
    (e)   *Stress tests:* remove catheter. Have patient cough and Valsalva in lithotomy and standing,
        if positive = SUI
    (f)   *Marshall test:* Repeat stress test with anatomic correction (i.e. tampons, examiner's fingers)

INCONTINENCE

NON-SURGICAL TREATMENT FOR INCONTINENCE

Treatment	Dosage/route of administration	Efficacy
Mechanical devices		
Absorbent materials	—	Useful
Pessaries	—	Useful
Bladder-neck support devices	—	Useful
Urethral plugs	—	Useful
Behavior modification		
Bladder drills and other pelvic-fploor exercises	—	Effective
Vaginal cones	—	Effective
Psychotherapy	—	Possibly effective
Hypnosis	—	No clinical data
Biofeedback	—	No clinical data
Acupuncture	—	No clinical data
Avoid bladder irritants	—	Ineffective
Electrical stimulation	—	Possibly effective
Pharmacologic treatment		
Anticholinergic drugs		
Methantheline bromide	50 mg p.o. q.i.d.	Effective
Propantheline bromide	15–30 mg p.o. q.i.d.	Effective
Emepronium bromide	200 mg p.o. t.i.d./q.i.d.	Probably effective
Emepronium carrageenate	300–500 mg p.o. q.i.d.	Probably effective
Scopolamine	0.5 mg q.d. transdermal	Probably effective
Fentonium bromide	20 mg p.o. t.i.d.	Possibly effective
Antispasmodic/spasmolytic drugs		
Flavoxate hydrochloride	200 mg p.o. q.i.d.	Minimally effective
Oxybutynin chloride	5–10 mg p.o. t.i.d.	Possibly effective
Dicyclomine hydrochloride	10–20 mg p.o. t.i.d./q.i.d.	Ineffective
Tricyclic antidepressants		
Imipramine hydrochloride	10–50 mg p.o. b.i.d.	Possibly effective
Doxepin	50–75 mg p.o. q.h.s.	Possibly effective
Calcium antagonists		
Terodiline hydrochloride	12.5–25 mg p.o. b.i.d.	Possibly effective
Nifedipine	1–20 mg p.o. b.i.d.	Possibly effective
Flunarizine	20 mg p.o. q.d.	Possibly effective
Prostaglandin synthetase inhibitors		
Flubiprofen	50 mg p.o. t.i.d./q.i.d.	Possibly effective
Indomethacin	50–100 mg p.o. b.i.d.	Minimally useful
Mefenamic acid	250–500 mg p.o. t.i.d.	Selectively useful
Muscarinic receptor antagonist		
Tolterodine tartrate	2 mg p.o. b.i.d.	Effective

Continued

Continued

Miscellaneous drugs

Baclofen	5 mg p.o. q.i.d.	Possibly effective
Bromocriptine	1–5 mg p.o. q.d.	Not effective
Terbutaline	5 mg p.o. t.i.d.	Possibly effective
Salbutamol	4 mg p.o. t.i.d.	Possibly effective
Prazosin	1–2 mg p.o. t.i.d.	Not effective
Mazindol	2–3 mg p.o. q.d.	Possibly effective
Lignocaine	Intravesical	Not effective
Propiverine hydrochloride	15 mg p.o. t.i.d.	Possibly effective

INCONTINENT PATIENT

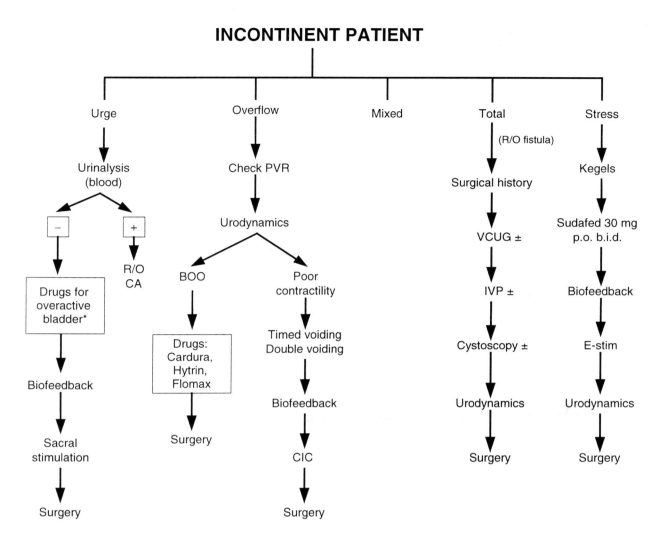

*Dicyclomine HCl 10-20 mg t.i.d.
Flavoxate HCl (Urispas) 100-200 mg t.i.d.
Imipramine HCl (Tofranil) 10-50 mg b.i.d.
Oxybutynin HCl (Ditropan) 2.5-5.0 mg t.i.d.-q.i.d.
Controlled-release oxybutynin (Ditropan XL) 5-20 mg q.d.
Propantheline bromide (Pro-Banthine) 15 mg t.i.d.
Tolterodine (Detrol) 2 mg b.i.d. + Pyridium Plus
(Pyridium 150 mg + hyocyamine HBr 0.3 mg + butabarbital 15 mg) one q.i.d.

INTERSTITIAL CYSTITIS (IC): DIAGNOSIS AND TREATMENT ALGORITHM

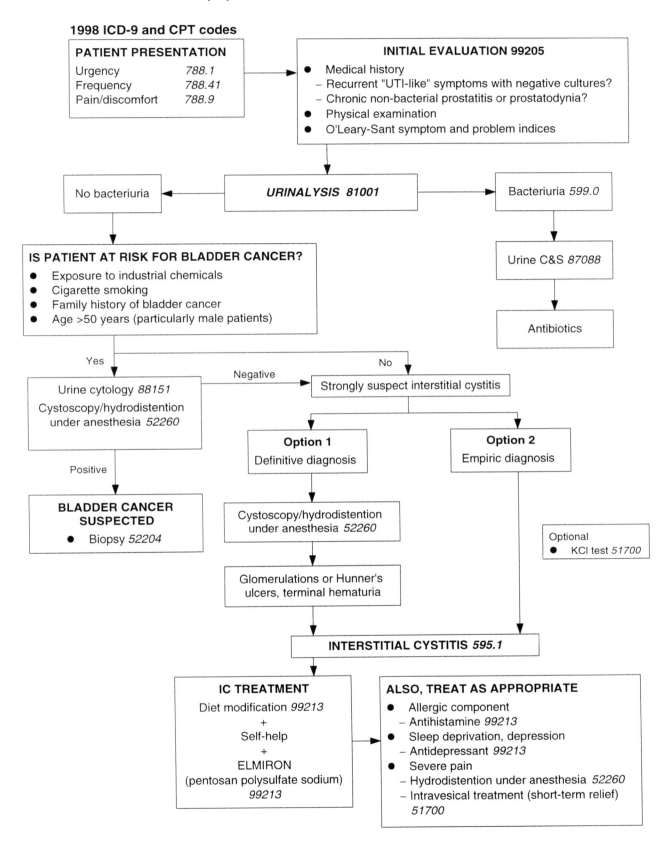

1998 ICD-9 and CPT codes

PATIENT PRESENTATION

Urgency	*788.1*
Frequency	*788.41*
Pain/discomfort	*788.9*

INITIAL EVALUATION 99205

- Medical history
  - Recurrent "UTI-like" symptoms with negative cultures?
  - Chronic non-bacterial prostatitis or prostatodynia?
- Physical examination
- O'Leary-Sant symptom and problem indices

URINALYSIS *81001*

No bacteriuria

Bacteriuria *599.0*

Urine C&S *87088*

Antibiotics

IS PATIENT AT RISK FOR BLADDER CANCER?

- Exposure to industrial chemicals
- Cigarette smoking
- Family history of bladder cancer
- Age >50 years (particularly male patients)

Yes

No

Urine cytology *88151*
Cystoscopy/hydrodistention under anesthesia *52260*

Negative → Strongly suspect interstitial cystitis

Positive

BLADDER CANCER SUSPECTED

- Biopsy *52204*

Option 1
Definitive diagnosis

Option 2
Empiric diagnosis

Optional
- KCl test *51700*

Cystoscopy/hydrodistention under anesthesia *52260*

Glomerulations or Hunner's ulcers, terminal hematuria

INTERSTITIAL CYSTITIS *595.1*

IC TREATMENT

Diet modification *99213*
+
Self-help
+
ELMIRON
(pentosan polysulfate sodium)
99213

ALSO, TREAT AS APPROPRIATE

- Allergic component
  - Antihistamine *99213*
- Sleep deprivation, depression
  - Antidepressant *99213*
- Severe pain
  - Hydrodistention under anesthesia *52260*
  - Intravesical treatment (short-term relief) *51700*

INFERTILITY

DEFINITION

Couples having unprotected intercourse for one year without successful conception. (Affects approximately 14% of American couples)

CAUSES

(1) **Male factor** (35%)
Prior testicular surgery; history of STD; post-pubertal mumps; genital radiation; chemotherapy; hypospadias; retrograde ejaculation; varicocele; exposure to: heat, toxic chemicals, drugs, alcohol

(2) **Pelvic factor** (25%)
History of PID; septic abortion; ruptured appendix; IUD; pelvic tuberculosis; endometriosis; ectopic pregnancy; adnexal surgery; leiomyomas or DES exposure

(3) **Ovulatory factor** (20%)
Secondary amenorrhea; oligomenorrhea; luteal phase defect; hyper/hypothyroidism; hirsutism; galactorrhea; hot flushes; weight loss; obesity; stress

(4) **Cervical factor** (10%)
History of cone biopsy; cautery; cervicitis; obstetric trauma; DES exposure

INITIAL EVALUATION

Thorough history

Medical, surgical, sexual, menstrual, obstetric, contraceptive, social, family and previous childbearing

Physical exam

Special attention to risk factors listed above

Diagnostic tests

Semen analysis (male factor); basal body cell temperature charting x3 months (ovulatory factor); postcoital test (cervical factor); consider HSG (pelvic factor)

ADDITIONAL EVALUATION/MANAGEMENT

Male factor

Urologic exam, serum testosterone, FSH, testicular biopsy, semen fructose, diabetes screen, sperm penetration assay

Treatment

Hypogonadism – hMG or GnRH
Varicocele – surgical ligation
Decreased penetration/oligospermia – IVF, ICSI

Pelvic factor

(1) **Tubal disorders**
HSG, laparoscopy
Treatment: tuboplasty/lysis of adhesions (laparoscopy), IVF

(2) **Uterine disorders**
HSG, ultrasound
Treatment: hysteroscopic lysis of adhesions/metroplasty/septoplasty (followed by ABX and high-dose E_2), myomectomy

(3) **Endometriosis**
Laparoscopy
Treatment: danazol/GnRH agonist (OCs), laparoscopic fulguration (mod/severe)

Ovulatory factor

FSH/LH, prolactin, thyroid profile, progesterone challenge, endometrial biopsy (luteal phase), serum progesterone, MRI (inc PRL)

Treatment: hyperprolactinemia – Parlodel

Positive progesterone challenge – Clomid; +/- dexamethasone;
+/– hCG

Failed Clomid – Pergonal (I&E specialist)

Luteal phase defect – progesterone suppositories 25 mg b.i.d.
(luteal phase – 10 wks)

Cervical factor

Spinnbarkeit, mucus amount, ferning, os patency

Culture – *Ureaplasma/Chlamydia*

Treatment: absent/poor quality mucus – IUI or low-dose E_2

Ureaplasma/Chlamydia – antibiotics

INFERTILITY

INTRAUTERINE INSEMINATION/TIMING OF OVULATION INDUCTION

Prerequisites

(1) Abnormal semen analysis
Normal semen: sperm count >20 million/ml
motility at least 50%
morphology at least 30%
leukocytes <1 million/ml

(2) Male should also have history/physical, endocrine work-up p.r.n., antisperm ab testing p.r.n., sperm function testing, or radiologic evaluation p.r.n.

(3) Female should have HSG, GC/*Chlamydia* cultures, postcoital test, and late luteal phase endometrial biopsy, laparoscopy and hysteroscopy may be indicated in some

(4) HIV & hepatitis tests should be considered initially for both partners

Timing

Prior to ovulation or at the time of; (**not** after ovulation)

LH kits, ultrasound, cervical mucous for Spinnbarkeit/ferning

Ovulation usually occurs 24–36 hrs after the LH surge

hCG 10,000 units – ovulation occurs 34–36 hrs after injection

Seminal wash

Mix with physiologic buffer (Hamm's) – centrifuge on low – pellet – resuspend by diluent. Use 0.5 ml for IUI (not too much volume *in* uterus). Best for patients with hypospadias, retrograde ejaculation, or pure oligospermia

(1) **Clomid**: 50 mg day 5–9 or day 3–7 (recruitment of more follicles)
Confirm ovulation with LH kit, BBT, U/S endo Bx, or mid-luteal phase serum progesterone
Increase by 50 mg/d p.r.n. subsequent cycle p.r.n.

(2) **hCG**: to be given 7 days after the last dose of CC or when ultrasound reveals a follicle of 22–24 mm diameter. No more than six ovulatory cycles recommended

(3) **Human menopausal gonadotropins**
Prior to giving hMG, U/S to rule out ovarian cysts; serum estradiol (E_2) on 3rd day of cycle
If no cysts >10 mm and E_2 [ ] <50 pg/ml, start

hMG 150 IU/d on day 3
Check E_2 levels on day 4, 6, and 8
Levels should be 100–200 (day 4), 400–600 (day 6), and 800–1200 pg/ml (day 8). Dosage adjusted accordingly
hCG 10,000 U IM when a single follicle or multiple follicles have reached 17 mm or > in diameter
hCG 5000 U IM or none given if concern about hyperstimulation

IUI performed at 34–36 hrs after hCG injection. Progesterone 250 mg IM or 25 mg supp b.i.d. started on day of IUI. Serum β-hCG level is obtained 16–18 days after IUI. IUIs timed at 18 and 42 hrs after hCG are superior to a single insemination

IUI

Insemi-Cath (Cook OB/GYN) on TB syringe or Mini Space IUI-Cath (1-800-441-1973)
0.2 ml of air then 0.5 ml   (to fundus)
No lubricants
Clean cervix with normal saline
Delay injection until no cramping
Pt to lie for 15 min after IUI (? Effectiveness)

Complications

Spontaneous abortion – 26% vs 10–15%
Ectopic   – increased to 8% vs 1%
Multiple pregnancies   (with hMG 25–30%)
                              (with CC   5–10%)
Ovarian hyperstimulation – 1% (especially if E_2 >2000)
IUI with hMG significantly increases pregnancy rates especially with men with impaired semen parameters
Refer to IVF or IVF with intracytoplasmic sperm injection if sperm counts <5 million/ml or linear progressive motility <20%

INTRAUTERINE GROWTH RESTRICTION (IUGR)

DEFINITION

In general, growth restriction is diagnosed when fetal weight falls below the 10th percentile of weight for gestational age. One or two standard deviation or more below the mean weight expected for a given gestational age

Before recognition and management of fetal growth restriction can be accomplished, the gestational age must be established. There are two types of IUGR:

(1) *Symmetric growth restriction* (20%) – occurs early in pregnancy and decreases the overall size of the fetus in weight and in length. It is most likely due to some significant maternal insult – such as malnutrition or infection or to fetal malformations, or chromosomal abnormalities

(2) *Asymmetric growth restriction* (80%) – results from some later insult that would tend to effect cellular hypertrophy, decrease subcutaneous fat and a decrease in abdominal circumference with preservation of head and femur growth. It is associated with maternal hypertension, renal disease, multiple gestation, etc.

ETIOLOGY OF IUGR

Maternal	Placental	Fetal
Pre-eclampsia	Abnormal presentation	Chromosomal abnormalities
Chronic hypertension	Chronic villitis	Multifactorial defects
Chronic renal disease	Placenta infarcts	Infections
Connective tissue disorder	Placenta hemangiomas	Multifetal pregnancies
Diabetes with vascular lesions	Placenta previa	
Sickle cell anemia	Circumvallate placenta	
Cardiac disease Class III or IV		
Severe malnutrition		
Smoking		
Alcohol ingestion		
Infection		

SCREENING AND DIAGNOSIS OF IUGR

Antepartum screening methods to detect IUGR fetus include:

(1) Careful serial measurement of uterine fundal height
(2) Progressive weight gain of the month
(3) Growth profile by ultrasound scanning

    (a) Progressive growth of biparietal diameter, fetal limb length, head circumference

    (b) Amniotic fluid volume
(Oligohydramnios is a common finding in IUGR) 90% of cases may be the earliest sign detected on ultrasound

(c) Head to abdominal circumference
HC/AC ratio in a normal growing fetus is:
  1 > before 32 wks
  1 = at 32 to 34 wks
  1 < after 34 wks

In fetus affected by asymmetric growth restriction, the HC remains larger than that of the body. The HC/AC ratio is then elevated

(d) Femur to abdomen ratio
Femur length is minimally affected by fetal growth impairment
Abdominal circumference which is the most affected measurement
FL/AC remains constant after 20 wks. FL/AC is 22 at all gestational ages from 21 wks to term
FL/AC ratio greater than 23.5 suggests IUGR

(e) Doppler wave form analysis. S/D ratio of umbilical artery. The development of Doppler ultrasound has provided the obstetrician with a new tool for the assessment of IUGR fetus

The researchers found that the negative predictive value of a normal S/D ratio (normal S/D <3) was 95%

The positive predictive value of an S/D ratio greater than 3.0 was 49%

An exciting possibility of Doppler examination is that it may be useful in making the critical distinction between the fetus that is small and healthy (SGA) and the one that is truly growth retarded. The majority of SGA babies have normal S/D ratio

Reversed end diastolic flow in the umbilical artery reflects severe fetal compromise and is an ominous finding. It is associated with 50–64% mortality rate, so delivery of the fetus is recommended when reversed end diastolic flow is detected

MANAGEMENT

Remote from term

(1) Intervention to improve intrauterine environment
(2) Avoid smoking, alcohol, drugs
(3) Control maternal disease
(4) Adequate maternal nutrition
(5) Decrease physical activity (bed rest)
(6) Fetal surveillance
  (a) NST
    Depending on the clinical circumstance the frequency of NST testing varies from once every week to every day
    Daily NSTs are indicated for patients with severe IUGR and with S/D ratios above 6
  (b) Contraction stress test (CST)
  (c) Biophysical profile (BPP)
    – (b) and (c) may be used to follow abnormal NSTs
    – delivery of the baby is the best management when the backup test suggests fetal compromise
  (d) Ultrasound every 2–3 wks for internal growth
  (e) Fluid volume
    This evaluation should be performed every week, and the frequency of NST testing should be increased if the amount of fluid decreases. Delivery may be indicated if severe oligohydramnios develops

Close to term or during delivery

(1) Close monitoring during labor
(2) Because of the high incidence of intrapartum asphyxia, labor and delivery in IUGR babies should be managed aggressively. The liberal use of Cesarean section is advised

(3)   Direct fetal monitoring using scalp electrode and uterine pressure catheter should be initiated as early as possible

(4)   Amnioinfusion should be performed early in labor if the amniotic fluid volume is decreased

(5)   Even mild signs of distress should be followed with scalp stimulation or fetal scalp pH sampling

(6)   The second stage of labor, with its well-known tendency toward low pH values, should be kept to a minimum (use of forceps or vacuum when the vertex is well below plus 2 station)

(7)   The best choice for pain relief during labor is epidural anesthesia

(8)   The placenta of an IUGR baby needs careful examination by a competent placental pathologist

(9)   Pediatrician should be present at the time of delivery

INTRAUTERINE GROWTH RESTRICTION - IUGR

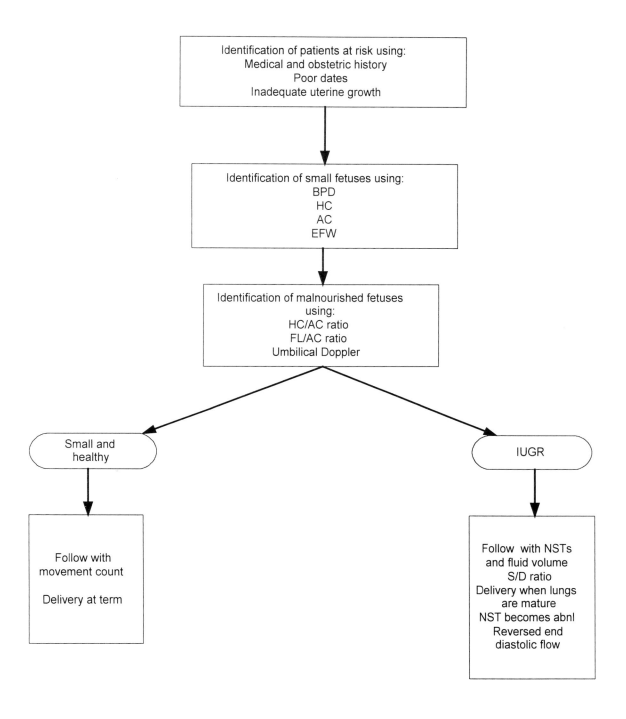

Identification of patients at risk using:
Medical and obstetric history
Poor dates
Inadequate uterine growth

Identification of small fetuses using:
BPD
HC
AC
EFW

Identification of malnourished fetuses using:
HC/AC ratio
FL/AC ratio
Umbilical Doppler

Small and healthy

IUGR

Follow with movement count

Delivery at term

Follow with NSTs and fluid volume
S/D ratio
Delivery when lungs are mature
NST becomes abnl
Reversed end diastolic flow

LABOR MEDICATIONS

IVFs

RL – better for pre-major conduction anesthesia
(Infusing any solution containing dextrose at high rates may result in osmotic diuresis and consequent dehydration)

PAIN

Sublimaze (Fentanyl) 1–2 cc IV q. 1–2 hrs p.r.n. pain
Demerol 50–100 mg, Phenergan 15–50 mg = IM every 3–4 hrs or dec dosages IV
Stadol 1 mg IV or 1–2 mg IM every 4 hrs
(Do not use if delivery anticipated within 4 hrs)
Nubain 5–20 mg IV or 10–20 mg IM every 2–4 hrs
(Maximum daily dose is 160 mg)

SEDATION

Nembutal 100–200 mg p.o.
Seconal 100–200 mg IM
Demerol 100 mg IM
Morphine 10 mg IM

ANTACID

30 ml of 0.3 M sodium citrate with citric acid (Bicitra) before anticipated general anesthesia to protect against aspiration pneumonitis

HYPERTENSION

Apresoline 5–10 mg IV bolus every 15–20 min until diastolic 90–100
Normodyne 20, 40, 80 mg then 80 mg thereafter at 10-min intervals (max of 300 mg)
Adalat, Procardia 10–20 mg p.o. every 20–30 min

RIPENING/AUGMENTATION

Prepidil Gel intracervical every 6–8 hrs no more than 3 in 24 hrs
Prostin 2.5 mg suppository intravaginal every 3–6 hrs
Cervidel tampon intravaginal 12–15 hrs prior to induction
Cytotech 25 µg intravaginal every 3–6 hrs
Pitocin 0.5–1 mIU/min with inc to 1–2 mIU/min at 30–60-min intervals
    2 mIU/min with inc to 2 mIU/min at 30–60-min intervals
    6 mU/min with inc to 6 mU/min at 20-min intervals

INDUCTION

'DrT' pitocin protocol

Augment: 1 mu/min IV then inc by 1 mu/min IV every 30 min
Active I: 6 mu/min IV and inc by 1 mu/min every 30 min

Active II: 6 mu/min IV and inc by 6 mu/min every 15 min
36 mu/min is maximum unless ordered to increase by MD

DIABETIC MANAGEMENT

Regular insulin 50 units in 500 ml of NS
Shake well – run out 50 ml waste to ensure absorption of surfaces
Continuous pump rate of 0.5 units/hr or > with increments of 0.5–1 unit/hr to obtain necessary glucose levels
Patient should also receive D5LR ml/hr to avoid starvation during labor
Check glucose values every hour with finger stick test strips
Adjust infusion p.r.n.

MASTALGIA

Mastalgia (mastodynia) is confined to the breast tissue and may be cyclic or non-cyclic and diffuse or localized. All women presenting with mastalgia deserve a complete evaluation including: breast-oriented history, complete breast examination, mammography (if over age 25), and fine-needle aspiration of any palpable dominant breast mass

If no significant abnormality is discovered, the patient can be reassured that there is no evidence of breast cancer and that her symptoms are common to many women – probably physiologic (end organ sensitivity)

Fewer than 15% of women with breast cancer present with pain as a chief complaint. Breast cancer pain is usually localized, non-cyclic and associated with a palpable mass

More than 75% of women presenting with mastalgia, after complete breast evaluation, will be satisfied with, and appropriately treated by reassurance. If further therapy is required, it should be tried in a step-wise fashion starting with:

(1) **Mechanical measures**: changing to a brassiere with good support, no wires, and no pressure points; heating pad or hot towels; massage
(2) **Physiological measures**: ventilation of any acute stress caused by exposure to breast cancer patients or information
(3) **Dietary measures**: weight reduction if obese; premenstrual salt restriction
(4) **Pharmacologic measures**:
    (a) 1/35 monophasic oral contraceptive therapy
    (b) Danazol – 100 mg twice a day until the mastalgia is controlled. In menstruating women, Danazol treatment should begin during menstruation to avoid the possibility of pregnancy, a contraindication to Danazol. The dose can be increased incrementally up to 400 mg a day

        After the breast symptoms have been controlled for at least a month, the dose of Danazol can often be reduced incrementally to as low as 50 mg per day. The patient should be maintained on the lowest effective dose for at least 6 months. As many as 50% of women will experience return of their mastalgia within 6 months after cessation of therapy. In these cases, Danazol therapy can be repeated

        Effective non-hormonal contraception should be practiced during Danazol treatment. Side-effects of treatment include: irregular menstrual bleeding and masculinization

MASTALGIA

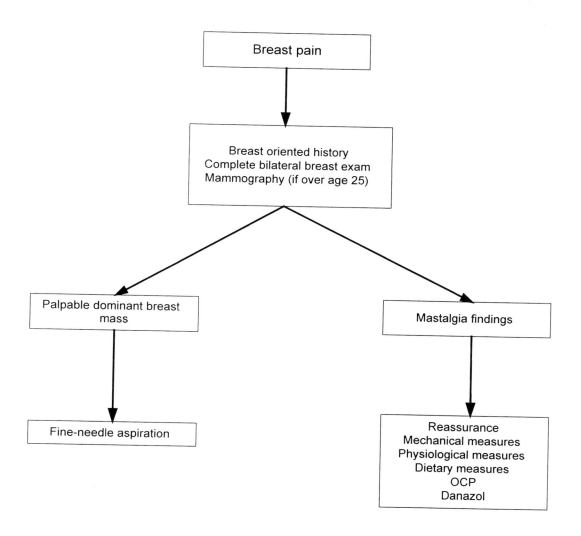

MEDICINES WITH COMMON DOSAGES

ANTIBIOTICS

Augmentin – 250 mg one tab p.o. t.i.d.

Ampicillin – 500 mg one tab p.o. q.i.d.

Doxycycline (Minocin, Doryx, or Monodox) – 100 mg one tab p.o. b.i.d. – *contraindicated in pregnancy*

Erythromycin – 250 mg one tab p.o. q.i.d., (**ERYC** 250 mg), or (**PCE** 500 mg b.i.d.)

Tetracycline – 250 mg *or* 500 mg p.o. q.i.d. – *contraindicated in pregnancy*

Metronidazole – 500 mg (**Flagyl** or **Satric**) p.o. b.i.d.

Floxin – 300 mg or 200 mg (see insert for different indications) – *contraindicated in pregnancy*

Bactrim DS *or* **Septra DS** one tab p.o. b.i.d.

Sulfamethoxazole – 500 mg one tab p.o. b.i.d.

Macrodantin – 50 mg or 100 mg p.o. t.i.d. or q.i.d.

Macrobid – 1 tab p.o. b.i.d.

Keflex – 250 mg or 500 mg p.o. q.i.d.

Ceclor – 250 mg one tab p.o. t.i.d.

Omniflox – 400 mg one tab p.o. daily (for non-complicated UTIs)

Cipro – 250 mg, 500 mg, or 750 mg p.o. b.i.d. – *contraindicated in pregnancy*

Biaxin – 500 mg p.o. b.i.d.

Zithromax – 250 mg two tabs p.o., then 1 tab p.o. q. daily x4 days (Z-pak as directed)

BOWELS

Constipation

Metamucil – two fiber wafers with 8 oz liquid
Pericolace – 100 mg p.o. b.i.d.
Ducolax suppository – b.i.d.

OB constipation

Increase water – 8 glasses per day
Bran cereal at night
Prune juice
Call back for stool softener p.r.n.

Traveler's diarrhea

Prevention: TMP 160 mg/SMX 800 mg → one DS tab p.o. daily or doxycycline 100 mg p.o. b.i.d. then daily

Treatment: Cipro 500 mg p.o. b.i.d.
Liperamide two tabs then one tab after each loose stool not to exceed 8 tabs per day
HYDRATION!

COUGHS/COLDS

Anatuss One tab p.o. q. 12 hrs for nasal congestion and dry cough

Anamine One tab p.o. b.i.d. or deconamine one tab p.o. b.i.d. for runny nose, sneezing, nasal congestion

Vitamin C 500–1000 mg daily

OPHTHALMOLOGICALS

Neosporin Ophth Sol. 10 cc 1–2 gtts. q. 2–3 hrs

Opthaine (local anesthesia) b.i.d.–q.i.d.

OTICS

Auralgan Otic Sol ½ oz 1gtt. q. 1–2 hrs till no pain
Debrox 1 oz 5–10 gtts. b.i.d. x3–4 days

PAIN

Morphine 8–10 mg IM or 2 mg IV or MS Contin 30 or 60 mg tabs p.o. q. 12 hrs
Ketorolac (Toradol) 30–60 mg IM then p.o. q. 6 hrs
Meperidine (Demerol) 25–75 mg IM or IV. Mepergan fortis p.o. q. 3–4 hrs
Sublimaze (Fentenyl) IV or transdermal 1–2 cc/hr
Oxycodone (various forms and brand names)
Dilaudid 1, 2, 3, or 4 mg IM, p.o., IV, or rectal suppositories
B+O suppositories (Professional Pharmacy, Dalton, Ga)

SEDATION

Halcion 0.25 mg–0.5 mg
Morphine 15 mg
Nembutal 100–200 mg
Placidyl 500 mg p.o. hs
Scopolamine gr 1/100, 2nd dose 1/200 (very seldom used any more)

STAT "DISASTER" MIX

Isoprel 1 cc
Atropine 2 cc (0.8 mg)
Neosynephrine 1 cc (10 mg)

All in 20 cc H_2O → Give 5 cc STAT IV for unknown type cardiac arrest. Last resort – otherwise do not attempt this mixture

MENOPAUSE WITH ERT

HORMONE REPLACEMENT THERAPIES

Active ingredients	Brand name	Strengths	Manufacturer*	Minimum dosage/day**
ESTROGENS				
17β-estradiol				
Oral	Estrace	0.5, 1, 2 mg	Westwood-Squibb	0.5 mg
Transdermal	Estraderm	0.05, 0.1 mg[1]	Novartis	0.05 mg
	Vivelle	0.0375, 0.05, 0.075, 0.1 mg[1]	Novartis	0.05 mg
	Menorest[3]	0.0375, 0.05, 0.075 mg[1]	Rhone-Poulenc-Rorer	0.05 mg
	FemPatch	0.05, 0.1 mg[1]	Parke-Davis	0.05 mg
	Climara	0.05, 0.1 mg[2]	Berlex	0.05 mg
	Alora	0.05, 0.75, 0.1 mg	Proctor & Gamble	0.05 mg
Estropipate	Ogen	0.625, 1.25, 2.5 mg	Pharmacia & Upjohn	0.625 mg
	Ortho-Est	0.625, 1.25 mg	Ortho	0.625 mg
Esterified estrogens	Estratab	0.3, 0.625, 1.25, 2.5 mg	Solvay	0.3 mg
	Menest	0.3, 0.625, 1.25, 2.5 mg	SmithKline Beecham	0.625 mg
Conjugated equine estrogens (CEE)	Premarin	0.3, 0.625, 0.9, 1.25, 2.5 mg	Wyeth-Ayerst	0.625 mg
	Cenestin	0.625, 0.9 mg	Duramed	0.625 mg
Ethinyl estradiol	Estinyl	0.02, 0.05, 0.5 mg	Schering	
Chlorotrianisene	Tace	12 mg	Hoechst Marion Roussel	12 mg
Estradiol pellets	N/A	25 mg	Pharmacy Center	
PROGESTOGENS				
Progestins				
Medroxyprogesterone acetate (MPA)	Provera	2.5, 5, 10 mg	Pharmacia & Upjohn	2.5–5 mg for continous combined, 5–10 mg for sequential
	Cycrin	2.5, 5, 10 mg	ESI Lederle	2.5–5 mg for continuous combined, 5–10 mg for sequential
	Amen	10 mg	Carnick	10 mg for sequential
Norethindrone	Norlutin	5 mg	Parke-Davis	2.5 mg
Norethindrone acetate	Norlutate	5 mg	Parke-Davis	2.5 mg
Progesterones				
Micronized	N/A	50, 100, 200 mg	Compounding companies	50–100 mg for continuous combined, 200 mg for sequential
TESTOSTERONES				
Testosterone pellets	N/A	75 mg	Barter Pharm. Co.	
Testosterone cypionate Estradiol cypionate IM	Depo-Testadiol	1 mg/q. wk	Upjohn	

Continued

Continued

Active ingredients	Brand name	Strengths	Manufacturer*	Minimum dosage/day**
COMBINED PRODUCTS				
	Prempro	0.625 mg CEE and 2.5 mg MPA	Wyeth-Ayerst	1 tablet
	Prempro	0.625 mg CEE and 5 mg MPA	Wyeth-Ayerst	1 tablet
	Femhrt	5 µg ethinyl estradiol and 1 mg norethindrone acetate	Parke-Davis	1 tablet
	Prefest	1 mg estradiol 0.09 mg norgestimate	Ortho-McNeil	1 tablet
	Premphase	0.625 mg CEE, w/ 5 mg MPA in last 14 tablets	Wyeth-Ayerst	1 tablet
	Estratest	0.625 mg esterified estrogens and 1.25 mg methyltestosterone (MT); 1.25 mg esterified estrogens and 2.5 mg MT	Solvay	1 tablet
Transdermal patch	CombiPatch[1]	Estradiol 0.05 mg daily norethindrone acetate 0.14 and 0.25 mg (9 mm) 0.14 mg norethindrone q.d. (16 mm) 0.25 mg norethindrone q.d.	Rhone-Poulenc-Rorer	
ALTERNATIVES				
Raloxifene	Evista	60 mg	Lilly	60 mg

KEY:
[1]Change patch twice weekly
[2]Change patch once weekly
[3]Not available in US
*Sample listing; others available
**Some minimum dosages not available

MENOPAUSE WITHOUT ERT

CONTRAINDICATIONS TO ERT

Absolute contraindications

Current breast cancer
Current endometrial cancer
Acute DVT or evolving thromboembolic event
Undiagnosed vaginal bleeding

Relative contraindications

History of breast cancer
History of endometrial cancer
History of DVT
Chronic liver disease
Endometriosis
History of CVA or recent MI
Pancreatic disease
Fibrocystic breast disease
Large fibroid uterus
Familial hyperlipidemia
Hepatic porphyria
Hypertension aggravated by estrogen
Migraines aggravated by estrogen

RISK FACTORS FOR OSTEOPOROSIS

Non-modifiable risk factors

Female sex
Age >65 years
Caucasian or Oriental race
Premature menopause (spontaneous or surgical)
History of an atraumatic fracture
Loss of height of >1 inch
Family history of osteoporosis
Chronic steroid therapy
Coexisting medical conditions
    Hyperparathyroidism
    Hyperthyroidism
    Malignancies (e.g., myeloma)
    Cushing's syndrome

Modifiable risk factors

History of smoking
Reduced weight for height
Excessive alcohol consumption
Excessive caffeine consumption
Lack of exercise
Diet deficient in calcium
Diet deficient in vitamin D
High-protein diet
Medications
    Prolonged heparin therapy
    Chronic steroid therapy

MENOPAUSE WITHOUT ERT

TREATMENT OF VASOMOTOR SYMPTOMS WITHOUT ESTROGEN

Treatment	Dosage/route of administration	Efficacy (vs. placebo)
Steroid hormones		
Progestins		
Depomedroxyprogesterone	150 mg IMI q. 3 months	Effective
Medroxyprogesterone	20 (10–80) mg p.o. q.d.	Effective
Megesterol acetate	20 mg p.o. b.i.d.	Effective
Androgens		
4-Hydroxyandrostenedione	250–500 mg IMI q. 1–2 wks	Possibly effective
Danazol	100 mg p.o. q.d.	Possibly effective
Synthetic steroids		
Org-OD-14 (tibolone)	2.5 mg p.o. q.d.	Probably effective
Non-steroidal medications		
Clonidine	0.05–0.15 mg p.c. or transdermal 200 μg q.d.	Probably effective
α-Methyldopa	250–500 mg p.o. b.i.d.	Probably effective
Bellergal-Retard	Variable	Insufficient data
β-Blockers	Variable	Not effective
Clomiphene citrate	50–150 mg p.o. q.d.	Not effective
Naloxone	22 μg/min IV	Not effective
Lofexidine	0.1–0.6 mg p.o. b.i.d.	Possibly effective
Veralipride	100 mg p.o. q.d.	Possibly effective
Environmental alteration		
Layered clothing	------------	No clinical data
Moderate exercise	------------	No clinical data
Avoidance of caffeine	------------	No clinical data
Avoidance of spicy foods	------------	No clinical data
Avoidance of alcohol	------------	No clinical data
Warm room	------------	No clinical data
Natural remedies		
Vitamin B, C, or E	Variable	No clinical data
Zinc	Variable	No clinical data
Bee pollen	------------	No clinical data
Cohash	------------	No clinical data
Ginseng tea	------------	No clinical data
Fenugreek	------------	No clinical data
Gotu kola	------------	No clinical data
Licorice root	------------	No clinical data
Wild yam root	------------	No clinical data

MENOPAUSE WITHOUT ERT

TREATMENT OF PSYCHOSEXUAL ISSUES WITHOUT ESTROGEN

Treatment	Dosage/route of administration	Efficacy
Pharmacologic treatment		
Androgens		
Methyltestosterone	2.5 mg p.o. q.d.	Possibly effective
Natural remedies		
Vitamin C	500 mg p.o. q.d./b.i.d.	No clinical data
Tryptophan	Variable	Possibly useful
Inositol	100 mg p.o. q.d.	No clinical data
Vitamin B_6	50–100 mg p.o. q.d.	No clinical data
Magnesium	Variable	No clinical data
Behavioral and/or psychological interventions	------------------	Probably ineffective

TREATMENT OF UROGENITAL ATROPHY WITHOUT ESTROGEN

Prevention	Dosage/route of administration	Efficacy
Continued sexual activity	---------------	Effective
Lubrication		
Water-based lubricants	---------------	Useful
Petroleum-based lubricants	---------------	Useful
Vegetable oils	---------------	Useful
Polycarbophil	---------------	Useful
Douching with yogurt	---------------	Probably ineffective
Pharmacologic therapy		
Tamoxifen	20–40 mg p.o. q.d.	Probably ineffective

MENOPAUSE WITHOUT ERT

PREVENTION AND TREATMENT OF CARDIOVASCULAR DISEASE WITHOUT ESTROGEN

	Dosage/route of administration	Efficacy
PREVENTION		
Environmental modification		
Smoking cessation	----------------------	Effective
Moderate physical exercise	----------------------	Effective
Control cholesterol	----------------------	Effective
Control hypertension	----------------------	Effective
Control diabetes	----------------------	Effective
Control weight	----------------------	Effective
Pharmacological treatment		
Aspirin	81–325 mg p.o. q.d.	Effective
Moderate alcohol consumption	Variable	Effective
Progesterone	10–15 g per day	Possibly effective
HMG-CoA reductase inhibitors	Variable	Possibly effective
Niacin	1–2 g p.o. t.i.d.	Possibly effective
Bile resins	Variable	Possibly effective
Natural remedies		
Antioxidant vitamins (vitamin E, vitamin C, β-carotene)	Variable	No clinical data
TREATMENT		
Pharmacological treatment		
Aspirin	81–325 mg p.o. q.d.	Effective
β-Blockers	Variable	Effective long-term
Calcium-channel blockers	Variable	Possibly effective
ACE inhibitors	Variable	Possibly effective
SERM (Evista)	60 mg p.o. q.d.	Effective
Surgery		
Conservative (angioplasty)	--------------	Effective
Radical (coronary bypass, transplantation)	--------------	Effective

MENOPAUSE WITHOUT ERT

PREVENTION OF OSTEOPOROSIS WITHOUT ESTROGEN

	Dosage/route of administration	Efficacy
Prevention		
Screening		
Bone mass index	----------	Useful
Environmental modification		
Smoking cessation	----------	Effective
Avoid alcohol excess	----------	Probably effective
Moderate exercise	----------	Effective
Dietary modification		
Vitamin D	800 IU p.o. q.d.	Effective
Pharmacologic treatment		
Agents that retard bone resorption		
Calcium	500–800 mg p.o. q.d. (elemental calcium)	Effective
Calcitonin	50 IU p.o. q.i.d.	Effective
Calcitriol	0.5–1 µg p.o. q.d.	Probably effective
Agents that promote bone formation		
Sodium fluoride	50–75 mg p.o. q.d.	Effective
Parathyroid hormone	40 µg sc q.d.	Probably effective
Anabolic steroids	Variable	Probably effective
Pharmacologic treatment		
Agents that retard bone resorption		
Calcium	1500 mg p.o. q.d. (elemental calcium)	Effective
Salmon calcitonin	50 U q.d./q.i.d. IV or intranasal (100 IU b.i.d.)	Possibly effective
Vitamin D analogues		
Calcitriol	0.25 µg p.o. q.d.	Possibly effective
Ergocalciferol	800 IU p.o. q.d.	Possibly effective
Cholecalciferol	800 IU (20 µg) p.o. q.d.	Possibly effective
Bisphosphonates		
Etidronate	200–400 mg p.o. q.d. x2 wks, 12 wks off	Effective
Alendronate (Fosamax)	5–20 mg p.o. q.d.	Effective
Tiludronate	Not determined	Under investigation
Residronate	Not determined	Under investigation
Pamidronate	Not determined	Under investigation
Progesterone	Variable	Possibly effective
Thiazide diuretics	Variable	Probably ineffective
Tamoxifen (Nolvadex)	20–40 mg p.o. q.d. (10 mg b.i.d.)	Probably ineffective

Continued

Continued

	Dosage/route of administration	Efficacy
Agents that promote bone formation		
Sodium fluoride	50–75 mg p.o. q.d.	Effective
Parathyroid hormone	40 µg sc q.d.	Probably effective
Growth factors	Variable	Probably ineffective
Anabolic steroids	Variable	Probably ineffective
Potassium bicarbonate	60–120 mmol p.o. q.d.	Possibly effective
Selective Estrogen Receptor Modulators (SERM)		
Raloxifene (Evista)	60 mg p.o. q.d.	Effective
Tamoxifen (Nolvadex)	20–40 mg p.o. q.d. (10 mg b.i.d.)	Probably ineffective

OCCUPATIONAL HAZARDS TO PREGNANCY

STRESSORS DURING PREGNANCY

(1)	Standing more than 3 hrs	Increase in prematurity; no effect on birth weight
(2)	Lifting more than 12 kg	No studies show any effect on birth weight or PTL
(3)	Strenuous work	Most studies show no effect on birth weight or PTL

PHYSICAL AGENTS

(1) **Heat**

≥38.9 °C Increases the rate of spontaneous abortions or birth defects (mostly neural tube)

Women with early hyperthermic episodes – counseled and AFP + U/S studies

(2) **Radiation**

Preimplantation "All or None" phenomenon

Greatest effect during late first and early second trimester

<5 rads – no intervention recommended

>5 rads – counsel; offer sonogram screen for microcephaly

(3) **Video display terminals**

No known effect. Increased CTS – place keypad

(4) **Chemicals**

See chart regarding "Developmentally toxic exposures in humans." If necessary, contact CDC in Atlanta, GA (404) 639-6300; fax (404) 639-6324

E-mail: lan8@atsdhs2.cm.cdc.gov

(5) **Hairstylists**

Minimize by use of gloves. Dermatitis. Mutagenic but not teratogenic. Minimize exposure in first trimester

(6) **Painters/artists**

Lead salts are of concern associated with increased spontaneous abortions, infant cognitive impairment, stillbirth rates in humans, CNS abnormalities. Women at risk should be monitored prior to conception. Lead [ ] >10 mg/ml – remove from exposure and consider chelation before pregnancy. No consensus how to manage after pregnancy (increased lead from bone stores and the chelating agent calcium edetate may be developmentally toxic, probably decreased zinc stores)

(7) **Solvent workers**

Ethylene glycol, toluene or gasoline, etc. similar to ETOH syndrome

An excess of MR, hypotonia, microcephaly

(8) **Pesticide workers**

Carbaryl and pentachlorophenol. Animal studies demonstrate impaired reproductive success or cause skeletal and body wall defects

If ethylene glycol, toluene, gasoline, carbaryl, or pentachlorophenol are suspected, blood or urine levels along with liver function tests can be obtained and if abnormal, increased fetal monitoring of fetal development is recommended

DEVELOPMENTALLY TOXIC EXPOSURES IN HUMANS

Aminopterin
Androgens
Angiotensin-converting
   enzyme inhibitors
Carbamazepine
Cigarette smoking
Cocaine
Coumarin anticoagulants
Cytomegalovirus
Diethylstilbestrol
Ethanol (≥1 drink/day)
Etretinate
Hyperthermia
Iodides
Ionizing radiation (>10 rads)

Isotretinoin
Lead
Lithium
Methimazole
Methyl mercury
Parvovirus B19
Penicillamine
Phenytoin
Radioiodine
Rubella
Syphilis
Tetracycline
Thalidomide
Toxoplasmosis
Trimethadione
Valproic acid
Varicella

OLIGOHYDRAMNIOS

OLIGOHYDRAMNIOS

Oligohydramnios is defined as an AFI of ≤5 cm
Dysmaturity syndrome – post-term gestational assessment with thick meconium, deep decels
AFI Marginal = 13x inc perinatal mortality (57/1000)
Severe oligohydramnios = 47x inc perinatal mortality (188/1000)
2nd trimester oligohydramnios = 43%; w/ lethal pulmonary hypoplasia = 33%
Anhydramnios (no fluid) = 88% lethal outcomes
Severe, long-standing oligohydramnios inhibits lung growth and promotes limb defects (club foot, arm contractures)

PRINCIPAL DIAGNOSIS WITH OLIGOHYDRAMNIOS

(1) PROM
(2) Placental insufficiency
    (a) Chronic abruption
    (b) Maternal hypertension
    (c) Placental crowding in multiple gestation
    (d) Autoimmune disease (lupus, antiphospholipid syndrome)
(3) Urinary tract anomaly
    (a) Polycystic or multicystic dysplastic kidneys
    (b) Renal agenesis
    (c) Ureteral or urethral obstruction
(1) Try to r/o ROM
(2) U/S fetal renal systems – do amnio if cystic kidneys and renal pelvic condition (assess with trisomy 21 + 18)
(3) R/o IUGR – abd circ legs behind head
    High vas resistance or uterine Doppler studies corroborate oligo due to placental insufficiency
    Hospitalize if diagnosed
    26–32 wks – amnio – mature? – deliver
(4) Consider pulmonary hypoplasia (lung area ratio should be >66%)

DIAGNOSTIC ADJUNCTS

Amnioinfusion – infection
Dye infusion to r/o membranes
Furosemide test to visualize fetal bladder

MANAGEMENT

Continual antepartem testing
    Inc rates of meconium; fetal distress and C/S
Intrapartum amnioinfusion – improved but over-distended uterus
Maternal hydration – effective
Amniotic fluid volume normally diminishes *after 35 weeks'* gestation
Postterm patients are *5 times* more likely to develop oligohydramnios in 3–4 days after a normal AFI, as compared to term patients. Therefore, postterm patients should have *semi*-weekly amniotic fluid volume assessment, with pockets <3 cm being considered normal

ONCOLOGY STAGING

CERVIX

0	CIS
I	Carcinoma strictly confined to cervix
IA	Ca if Cx dxned by microscopy
IA1	Ca of Cx with minimal microscopic stromal invasion
IA2	Ca of Cx that are microscopically measured but no more than 5 mm in depth and no more than 7 mm in horizontal spread
IB	Lesions greater than those in IA2 whether seen clinically or not
II	Ca involves vagina but not as far as the lower third
IIA	No obvious parametrial involvement
IIB	Obvious parametrial involvement
III	Ca involves the lower third of the vagina
IIIA	No extension to the pelvic wall
IIIB	Extension to the pelvic wall and/or hydronephrosis or nonfunctioning kidney
IV	Ca extended beyond the true pelvis or involved the mucosa of bladder or rectum
IVA	Spread of the growth to adjacent organs
IVB	Spread to distant organs

OVARY

I	Growth limited to ovaries
IA	One ovary. No ascites. Capsule intact. No tumor on external surface
IB	Two ovaries. No ascites. Capsule intact. No tumor on external surface
IC	One or two ovaries but with ascites (+), capsule ruptured, or with tumor on external surfaces
II	Pelvic extension
IIA	Extension or metastases to uterus and/or tubes
IIB	Extension to other pelvic structures
IIC	IIA or IIB but with ascites, capsule ruptured, or with tumor on external surface of one or both
III	Positive nodes and/or implants outside pelvis
IIIA	Negative nodes but with microscopic seeding of peritoneal surfaces
IIIB	Negative nodes but with seeding of the peritoneal surfaces none exceeding 2 cm
IIIC	Positive nodes and/or seeding of the peritoneal surfaces exceeding 2 cm
IV	Distant metastasis

UTERUS

I	Confined to uterus	G1 = 5% nonsquamous etc growth
IA	Endometrium	G2= 6–50%
IB	Less than ½ the myometrium	G3 = more than 50% solid gr.pat.
IC	More than ½ the myometrium	
II	Spread to cervix	
IIA	Endocervical glandular involvement only	
IIB	Cervical stromal invasion	
IIIA	Invades serosa and/or adnexa and/or positive peritoneal cytology	
IIIB	Vaginal metastasis	
IIIC	Metastases to pelvic and/or para-aortic lymph nodes	

IVA   Tumor invasion of bladder and/or bowel mucosa
IVB   Distant metastases including intra-abdominal and/or inguinal lymph nodes

VULVA

0   CIS; intraepithelial carcinoma

I   Confined to vulva and/or perineum – 2 cm or less, no palpable nodes

II   Confined to vulva and/or perineum – more than 2 cm, no palpable nodes

III   Tumor of any size but with adjacent spread to lower urethra, and/or vagina and/or the anus, and/or unilateral regional lymph node metastasis

IVA   Invades urethra, bladder mucosa, rectal mucosa, pelvic bone, and/or bilat. node mets
IVB   Distant metastasis including pelvic lymph nodes

VAGINA

0   CIS, intraepithelial carcinoma

I   Vaginal wall

II   Subvaginal tissue but not extended to pelvic wall

III   Extension to the pelvic wall (including pubic bone)

IVA   Extension beyond the true pelvis or involves the bladder or rectum
IVB   Distant metastasis

FALLOPIAN TUBE

0   CIS (limited to tubal mucosa)

I   Limited to Fallopian tubes (IA, IB (both), and IC-ext onto or thru serosa + washings)

II   Pelvic extension (IIA to uterus +/or ovaries, IIB other, IIC – ext with + washings)

IIIA Microscopic mets outside pelvis; IIIB, less than 2 cm; IIIC, more than 2 cm +/or + n

IV   Distant mets

ONCOLOGY STAGING

OVARIAN CANCER

Origin	Name	Histogenesis	Unique finding	% Malignant
Coelomic epithelial • 80–85% of all ovarian tumors • Age at diagnosis older than 40 years	Serous	Ciliated tubal epithelium	Psammoma bodies; Tumor marker: CA-125	20%
	Mucinous	Columnar endocervical epithelium	Pseudomyxoma peritonei; Tumor marker: CEA	15%
	Endometrioid	Endometrial glands	Tumor marker: CA-125	95%
	Clear cell	Mesonephric tissue	Tumor marker: CA-125	98%
	Brenners	Transitional urothelium	Walthard cell rests	2%
Germ cell • 10–15% of all ovarian tumors • Age at diagnosis younger than 30 years	Teratoma mature	Many mature cell types	Rokitansky prominence	0–1%
	Teratoma immature	Fetal embryonic tissue	Tumor markers: α-FP, CA-125	100%
	Dysgerminoma	Primitive germ cells	Tumor marker: LDH	100%
	Gonadoblastoma	Dysgenetic gonads with Y chromosomes	Malignant only if there are associated dysgerminoma elements	0%
	Endodermal sinus	Extraembryonic tissue	Schiller–Duval bodies; Tumor marker: α-FP	100%
	Embryonal carcinoma	Embryonic tissue	Tumor markers: α-FP, β-hCG	100%
	Nongestational choriocarcinoma	Extraembryonic tissue	Tumor marker: β-hCG	100%
Gonadal–stromal • 3–5% of all tumors • Age at diagnosis 50 years, with a range of 20–80 years	Granulosa cell	Ovarian gonadal cells	Cal-Exner bodies; estrogen production; inhibin	<5%
	Fibroma	Thecoma elements	Seen with Meigs' syndrome	<5%
	Thecoma	Thecoma elements	Estrogen production	<5%
	Sertoli–Leydig cell	Testicular gonadal cells	Crystals of Reinke; testosterone production	<5%
	Lipid cell	Gonadal–stromal cells	Testosterone production	30%
	Gynandroblastoma	Both ovarian and testicular cell tissues	Testosterone production	100%

OSTEOPOROSIS

SYSTEMIC SKELETAL DISEASE

(1) Decreased bone mass
(2) Deterioration of bone architecture
(3) Increased bone fragility
(4) Increased susceptibility to fracture
(5) Relative increase in osteoclast to osteoblast activity

Risk factors

Estrogen deficiency/aging leading factors
- Hypoestrogenism (untreated menopause/oophorectomy/amenorrhea)
- Positive family history
- Caucasian/Asian race
- Small skeletal frame
- Tobacco use
- Sedentary lifestyle
- Alcohol use, greater than 3 drinks per week
- Prolonged steroid use

Diagnosis

(1) Careful history (risk factors, h/o "low trauma" fracture)
(2) Review differential diagnosis (hyperparathyroidism, renal failure, Paget's disease)
(3) Laboratory studies:

BONE DISORDER

	Osteoporosis	*Osteomalacia*	*Hyperpara-thyroidism*	*Renal failure osteodystrophy*	*Paget's disease*
Serum calcium	Normal	↓	↑	↓	Normal
Serum phosphorus	Normal	↓	↓	↑	Normal
Alkaline phosphatase	Normal	↑	↑	↑	⇑

(4) Bone densitometry (at-risk women not taking estrogen)
   (a) T-score = Standard deviation from mean peak bone mass
   (b) Osteopenia – T-score = – 1 to –2.5
   (c) Osteoporosis – T-score = < –2.5
   (d) Each 1 standard deviation decrease = 2–3x increase risk of fracture

Treatment

(1) *Estrogen therapy* (decreased osteoclast activity; decreased bone loss; decreased hip/spine fracture
**Flexible dosing (0.3–1.25 mg conjugated estrogens/0.5–2 mg micronized E_2)
Continuous (estrogen 0.625 mg/medroxyprogesterone 2.5 mg q.d.)
Cyclic (estrogen 0.625 mg D1-25/medroxyprogesterone 5 mg D16–25)
Progestin not necessary if uterus absent

(2) *Alendronate/calcitonin* (for patients who decline estrogen)
    (a)   Alendronate (decreased osteoclast activity/increased bone density)
            Prevention — 5 mg q.d. taken with water (8 oz) in a.m.
            Treatment — 10 mg q.d. taken with water (8 oz) in a.m.
    (b)   Calcitonin (decreased osteoclast activity/increased bone mass)
            200 IU intranasal spray q.d. (alternate nostrils)

(3) *Newer agents* (Raloxifene/Tibolone)
    (a)   Raloxifene–estrogen agonist (bone/liver) antagonist (endometrium/breast/CNS)
            30–150 mg q.d. (+500 mg q.d. calcium supplement)
    (b)   Tibolone-synthetic progestin (androgenic/'estrogenic' effects)
            1.25–2.5 mg q.d.

(4) *Supplements* (calcium/vitamin D)
    (a)   Calcium (maximum intake should not exceed 2500 mg)
            (calcium citrate is more soluble and better absorbed than calcium carbonate)

Age	*RDA*	
0–6 months	210 mg	
6–12 months	270 mg	
1–3 years	500 mg	
4–8 years	800 mg	
9–18 years	1300 mg	(same amt in pregnancy/
19–50 years	1000 mg	lactation)
51+ years	1200 mg	(1500 mg if not on ERT)

    (b)   Vitamin D (400–800 IU q.d.)

(5) Exercise (weight-bearing)
20–30 minutes per day at least 5 days per week. Exercise stimulates osteoblasts to form new bone

OSTEOPOROSIS TREATMENT ALGORITHM

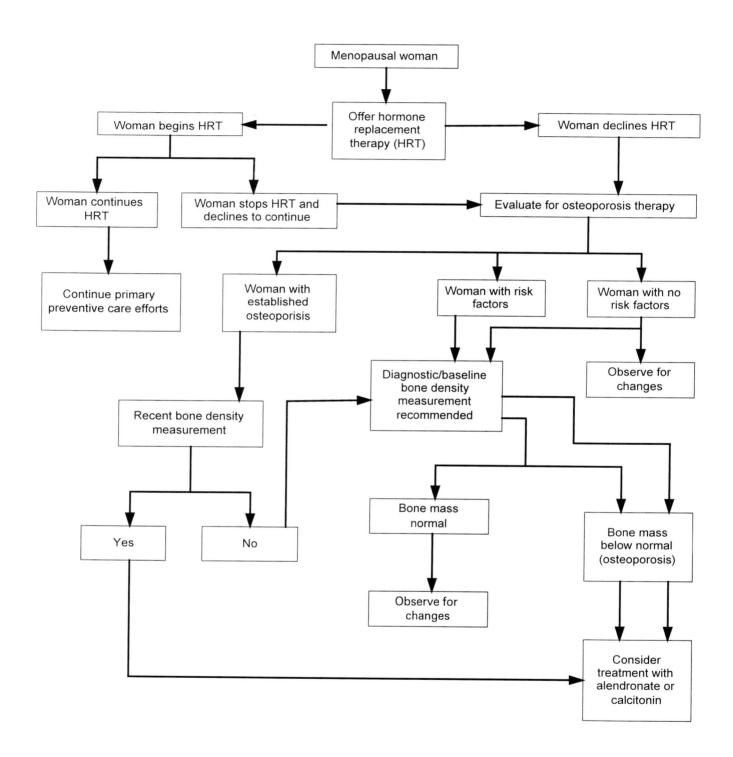

PAIN MANAGEMENT (CHRONIC)

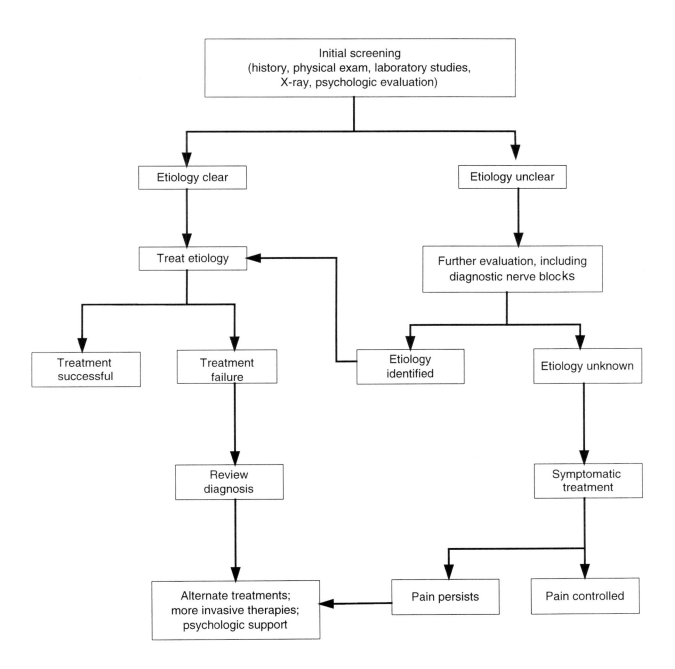

PAP SMEARS

PAP SCREENING

(*High-Risk Group*)

1 year– sexually active
  – h/o sexual activity
  – 18 years old
  – h/o HPV/HIV
  – smoking
  – multiple sexual partners

(*Low-Risk Group*)

1–3 years – monogamous
  – previous hysterectomy
  – three consecutive normal Paps

ABNORMAL PAPs

Benign cellular changes

Inflammation – treat organism – repeat Pap w/ cultures in 3–4 months (cultures w/ Pap?)

Reactive changes associated with:
  – inflammation   Treat with antibiotics/estradiol; repeat Pap in 3–4 months
  – atrophy
  – radiation
  – IUD

EPITHELIAL CELL ABNORMALITIES

Squamous dysplasia

ASCUS screening)	1st:	Repeat Pap 3–4 months x2 (if two consecutive within normal limits – annual
	2nd:	In absence of diagnosis intervention – colpo
LGSIL screening)	1st:	Repeat 3–4 months x2 (if two consecutive within normal limits – annual
	2nd:	Colpo
HGSIL SCCA	(Mod or severe) – colpo (if pregnant 1–2 wks)	

Glandular cell

Endometrial cells (benign)	– premenopausal	– regular screening
	– postmenopausal	– endometrial biopsy/D&C
AGUS	– colpo	– +/– endometrial biopsy
Adeno CA	– endocervical	
	– endometrial	

COLPOSCOPY

Cultures
Pap
ECC (Deferred in pregnancy – colpo + Pap every 3 months)
Directed biopsy (If possible deferred in pregnancy – colpo + Pap every 3 months)

Treatment – biopsy confirmed diagnosis

LSIL	– cryo
HSIL	– LEEP
	– CKC
+ECC	– CKC

After-treatment follow-up

Pap every 3–4 months until three consecutive within normal limits; then screening Paps
If abnormal, revert to abnormal Pap pathway

SCREENING PAP SMEARS

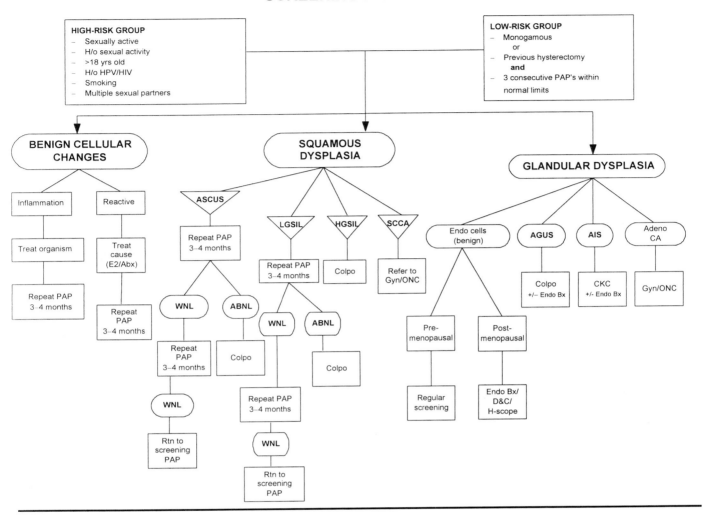

COLPOSCOPY

- Cultures
- PAP
- ECC — (Deferred in pregnancy/colpo + PAP q. 3 months)
- Directed Bx (Deferred in pregnancy/colpo + PAP q. 3 months)

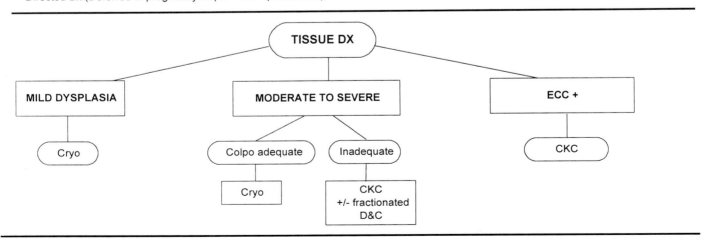

AFTER-TREATMENT FOLLOW-UP

- PAP q. 3 –4 months until three consecutive within normal limits; then screening PAPs
- If abnormal, revert to abnormal PAP pathway

PARASITOLOGIC INFECTIONS IN PREGNANCY

Infection	Organism	Symptoms	Route of infection	Diagnoses	Pregnancy effects	Placental trans	Drug of choice (FDA)	Alternate drug	Drug (if not pregnant)
Giardiasis	Giardia lamblia	Watery, bulky diarrhea; abd pain; flatulence; nausea, wt loss; malaise	Fecal–oral	Trophozoites in stool	Secondary maternal disease	None	Humatin (paromomycin) 30 mg/kg/day in 3 doses for 5–10 days (B)	Flagyl (metronidazole) 250 mg t.i.d. x5d (B) (last two trimesters)	AtabrineHCl (quinacrine) 100 mg/d x5 days (C)
Pinworms	Enterobius vermicularis	Intense perineal and anal itching particularly at night	Auto-inoculation	Demonstration of worms on adhesive tape	None known	None	Animinth, Conbantrin (pyrantel pamoate) 10 mg/kg – max 1 g (base) after 1st trimester Repeat dose 2wks later. Clothing/bedding to be washed in hot water and chlorine bleach		Vermox (mebendazole) Equizole Mentezol Thibenzole (thiabendazole)
Hookworms	Ancylostoma duodenate Necator americanus	Anemia	Skin penetration of larvae from soil	Eggs in fecal smears	Secondary to maternal anemia	None	Iron Pyrantel 11 mg/kg x3 days		
Amebiasis	Entamoeba histolytica	Asymptomatic or 10–50% Sxs of colicky lower abd pain	Fecal–oral	E. histolitica in stool or sigmoidoscopy	Secondary to maternal disease	None	Humatin 30 mg/kg/day in 3 doses x7 days. Give Flagyl 750 mg p.o. t.i.d. x10 days then Humatin for severe infections	If severe, give dehydro-emetine 1.5 mg/kg/day x5d CDC (404) 6393670	Iodoquinol or emetine
Malaria	Plasmodium ovale vivax Nonresistant P. falciparum Chloroquine-resistant P. falciparum	High fever/chills, abd pain, nausea vomiting, delirium	Anopheline mosquito	Plasmodium parasites in stained peripheral blood smears	Secondary to maternal disease	1–4% congenital malaria documented	Aralen (chloroquine) 1g then 500 mg at 6, 24, and 48 hrs then weekly till after delivery; then primaquine 15 mg daily x14 days post-partum (screen for G-6PD)	Parental quinine gluconate for life-threatening infections P. falciparum Rx for resistant P. falciparum is quinine 650 mg t.i.d. x3–7 days plus pyrimethamine/sulfadoxine, 3 tabs on day 3 of tx.	Larium (mefloquine
Pediculosis pubis (Crab louse)	Phthirius pubis	Pruritus and itching	Close contact usually sexual	Visualization of adult lice or nits (eggs) under magnification		None	Permethrine 1% Cream applied x10 min then washed off	Pyrethrines Piperonyl butoxide x10 min then washed off	Lindane 1% x4 min then wash

PELVIC INFLAMMATORY DISEASE (PID)

RISK FACTORS FOR PID

Age 14–24
Sexually active
Multiple sex partners
New sex partner
Hx of STD
Hx of PID
Use of an IUD for contraception
Nulliparity
Onset of pain during or within 1 wk of menses
Cigarette, alcohol or illicit drug use
Pelvic instrumentation

CRITERIA FOR CLINICAL DIAGNOSIS OF PID

Minimum criteria for clinical Dx (all three must be present)
Lower abdominal tenderness
Bilateral adnexal tenderness
Cervical motion tenderness
Additional criteria useful in Dx (one or more necessary for dx)
Oral temp >101 ˚F (>38.3 ˚C)
Abnormal cervical or vaginal discharge
Elevated ESR or C-reactive protein
WBC >10,500
Evidence of cervical infection with *Neisseria gonorrhea* or *Chlamydia trachomatis*
Tubo-ovarian abscess on sonography or radiologic test
Laparoscopic abnormalities consistent with PID
Histopathologic evidence on endometrial biopsy
CDC criteria for hospital admission
Adolescent patient
Concurrent HIV infection
Dx of PID uncertain
Failure of outpatient treatment
Inability of patient to follow or tolerate outpatient regimen
Inability to exclude surgical emergency
Pregnancy
Severe illness or nausea and vomiting
Suspected pelvic abscess
Uncertainty about clinical f/u within 24 hrs of starting antibiotic tx
All nulliparous women

PELVIC INFLAMMATORY DISEASE (PID)

IN-PATIENT TREATMENT GUIDELINES

Regimen A

Cefoxitin sodium (Mefoxin), 2 g IV q. 6 hr
        OR
Cefotetan disodium (Cefotan), 2 g IV q. 12 hr
        PLUS
Doxycycline 100 mg IV (Vibramycin IV) q. 12 hr
- continue this regimen for at least 48 hrs after clinical improvement
- after discharge, the patient continues doxycycline 100 mg p.o. b.i.d. for a total of 14 days

Regimen B

Clindamycin 900 mg IV q. 8 hr
        PLUS
Gentamicin in IV or IM (loading dose of 2 mg/kg of body weight followed by a maintenance dose of 1.5 mg/kg q. 8 hr
- continue this regimen for at least 48 hrs after clinical improvement
- after discharge, the pt is given doxycycline 100 mg p.o. b.i.d. or clindamycin 450 mg p.o. q.i.d. for 14 days

OUT-PATIENT TREATMENT GUIDELINES

Regimen A

Cefoxitin 2 g IM; plus Probenecid (Benemid), 1 g p.o. concurrently
        OR
Ceftriaxone (Rocephin), 250 mg IM
        PLUS
Doxycycline 100 mg p.o. b.i.d. for 14 days or Zithromax 1 g p.o.

Regimen B

Ofloxacin 400 mg p.o. b.i.d. for 14 days
        PLUS
Clindamycin 450 mg p.o. q.i.d. for 14 days
        OR
Metronidazole 500 mg p.o. b.i.d. for 14 days

PELVIC MUSCLE EXERCISE (PME)

PELVIC FLOOR EXERCISE (KEGEL EXERCISES)

66% Incidence of reduction during 16 week PME protocol, 2 months or longer

Written or verbal instructions usually inadequate

Errors in technique – contraction of auxiliary muscles (gluteal, thigh) and most seriously – a Valsalva or straining down effort

Audio tape: HELP for Incontinent People

   1-800-252-3337

30–80 per day with 10 second relaxation recommended between contractions

Quick "flick," "pull," "squeeze," "tighten," "lift," "clench," "contract"

Cones can be purchased to help train pelvic floor

FOLLOW-UP: Absence of gluteal or thigh contractions. Digital palpation of pelvic floor during PME – descent of clitoris and inward/up motion of anus – lifting of exam finger by three layers of perivaginal muscle layers

PELVIC MUSCLE EXERCISE

PATIENT GUIDE TO PREVENTION OR TREATMENT OF URINARY INCONTINENCE

Q   **What is pelvic muscle exercise?**

A   Pelvic muscle exercise (also called Kegel exercise) is the tightening and relaxing of the muscles that support the uterus, bladder, and other pelvic organs. Strong pelvic muscles can help prevent accidental urine leakage

Q   **Why should I do pelvic muscle exercise?**

A   Regular pelvic muscle exercise makes these muscles stronger. Women who have a problem with urine leakage have been able to eliminate or greatly improve this problem just by doing pelvic muscle exercise every day

Q   **How do I do pelvic muscle exercise?**

A   The feeling you should have when you are doing pelvic muscle exercise is that all the pelvic muscles are drawing inward and upward. A good way to learn the exercise is to pretend that you are trying to avoid the embarrassing passing of intestinal gas. Think about the muscles that tighten (or contract) to keep the gas from escaping. Bring that same tightening forward to the muscles around your vagina, and move the contraction up to the higher levels of your pelvis. There are three layers of muscle to tighten, and you can feel them as you move the contraction up to the highest level

IMPORTANT TIPS

(1)   Each contraction should be as hard or intense as you can make it without tightening your thigh or buttock muscles

(2)   Work up to holding each contraction for 2 seconds, then for 4, 6, 8, and 10 seconds as your muscles become stronger

(3)   Rest for at least 10 seconds (longer if you need to) between each contraction, so that each one is as hard as you can make it

(4)   Each contraction should reach the highest level of your pelvis; you will feel the pulling up and in over the three distinct layers of muscle

Q   **How often should I do these exercises, and how many should I do?**

A   If you have some problem with urine leakage, we recommend 30 contractions each day. You can expect to see some improvement after doing regular pelvic muscle exercise for about 6–8 wks, so don't be discouraged if you don't notice results right away. Remembering to contract the muscles prior to coughing, blowing your nose, or sneezing will help you avoid leakage. This technique can also help to control sudden urges to urinate

Q   Are there any mistakes to avoid with pelvic muscle exercise?

A   The most serious mistake is to strain down instead of drawing the muscles up and in. Trying this will show you what NOT to do: take a breath, hold it, and push down with your abdomen. You can feel a pushing out around your vagina. It is very important to avoid this straining down. To keep from straining down while you do pelvic muscle exercise, exhale gently and keep your mouth open each time you tighten the pelvic muscles. You can also keep your hands on your abdomen while you tighten your pelvic muscles. If you feel your stomach pushing out against your hands, you are straining down. Do not continue with pelvic muscle exercise until you check with your physician to learn how to do it properly

Avoid tightening thigh and buttock muscles. This takes away from the effectiveness of your pelvic muscle exercise. If it seems impossible not to tighten the thigh and buttock muscles, concentrate first on full relaxation, and then try gentle "flicks" of the pelvic muscles; for example, "flick, relax, flick, relax." After gaining confidence, try a second flick on top of the first, and then a third – "flick flick, flick, relax" – working the muscles to higher layers with each flick

KEYS TO SUCCESS

It is a challenge to work any new health habit into your everyday life. Here are some things that other women have found helpful in making pelvic muscle exercise a regular part of their self-care:

(1) Think about your usual day, and pick a time (about 15 min) when you will be able to do your pelvic muscle exercise every day. Maybe when you first wake up is a good time, or maybe afternoon or evening is better

(2) Decide on a way to remind yourself to do pelvic muscle exercise. You might put a note on your bathroom mirror, or plan to do your exercises during a TV program that you watch every day. Just think of something that happens every day that will remind you to do it

(3) Reward yourself for exercising each time you do it. You might get some special small candies and treat yourself to one each day that you remember to do pelvic muscle exercise. Or you could draw a small flower on your calendar to mark each day you exercise, and get yourself a real bouquet of flowers when you have drawn 10 flowers. Any small reward that you know will keep you working on this new habit is fine

(4) Monitor your progress, especially if you have a problem with urine leakage. You might want to keep a daily diary of whether you have had an accident and how many times it happened. Over the weeks, you will be able to measure your own progress. Another way is to see whether you can slow or stop your urine stream when you are going to the bathroom. We recommend that you try this no more than once a week. As your pelvic muscles get stronger, you will be able to stop the stream more quickly

Good luck on your program of pelvic muscle exercise! Please call your physician if you have any questions about this program to strengthen your pelvic muscles

PERIMENOPAUSAL BLEEDING

WHEN PATIENT IS NO LONGER OVULATING

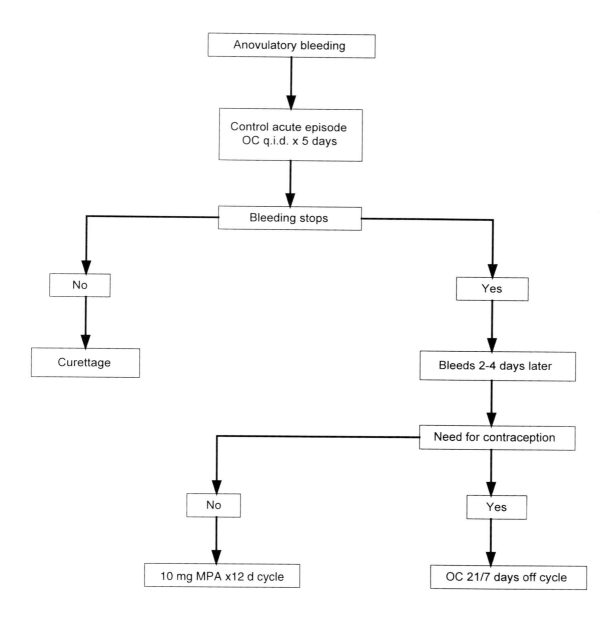

PERIMENOPAUSAL BLEEDING

PATIENT WHO IS TAKING HRT

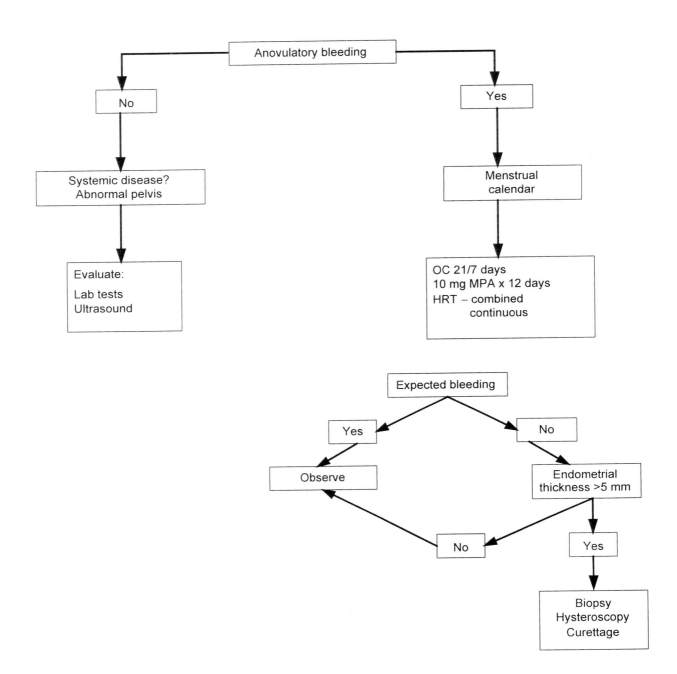

PLACENTA PREVIA

DEFINITION

A placenta previa is a placenta implanted on the lower uterine segment that prevents descent of the fetus. The degree to which the internal cervical os is covered by the placenta determines whether a placenta previa is classified as marginal, partial or complete:

(1) Complete: implantation of the placenta across the cervical os
(2) Partial: placenta covers part of internal os
(3) Marginal: placenta just reaches the edge of the internal os

PRE-DISPOSING FACTORS

(1) Advanced maternal age
(2) Increased parity
(3) Previous uterine surgery

SYMPTOMS

A placenta previa usually manifests its presence in the second trimester by painless vaginal bleeding. Another small percentage manifests for the first time at term

DIAGNOSIS

Obstetric ultrasound is the method of choice

MANAGEMENT

(1) Do not perform a pelvic examination until ultrasound report is available
(2) If a previa has been ruled out, the following steps should be taken:
    (a) Do speculum exam to rule out causes of bleeding such as cervicitis, polyps or cervical lesions
    (b) Look for other placental abnormalities such as placenta abruption
(3) If a placenta previa is diagnosed in second trimester, the following steps should be taken:
    (a) Start intravenous infusion of fluid with 18-gauge needle
    (b) Obtain a coagulation profile
    (c) Evaluate fetal viability, advanced labor or uncontrollable hemorrhage
       – If ultrasound examination shows no heart activity, consider termination. If fetus is alive, manage conservative (if bleeding is mild to moderate)
       – If advanced labor or uncontrollable bleeding is present, proceed with C/S
(4) Do not do a double set-up examination unless ready to commit to delivery
(5) Use of tocolytic agents:
    (a) Use only when the uterus is contracting and/or vaginal bleeding is not sufficient to cause maternal hypotension
    (b) Do not use if blood replacement would be unable to keep up with blood loss or the patient is in active labor
(6) Provide patient with risk, benefits and alternatives regarding increased incidence of intrauterine growth restriction, need for adequate nutrition, and cessation of smoking
(7) Repeat ultrasound examination at 35–36 wks

PLACENTA PREVIA

If placenta previa is diagnosed at 35–36 wks, the following steps should be taken:
(1) Complete previa
    (a) Determine fetal lung maturity (PG or L/S ratio) via ultrasound-guided amniocentesis
    (b) If fetal lungs mature, delivery by C-section
    (c) If fetal lungs immature, monitor weekly for maturity, then do C-section
(2) Marginal or partial previa
    (a) Do amniocentesis as above
    (b) If fetal lungs mature, consider two possible causes:
       – Double set-up when ready to commit to delivery
       – Follow with serial ultrasound to see whether placenta moves upward, as long as there is no further bleeding
    (c) If no longer a placenta previa on ultrasound, treat as a normal pregnancy

POLYHYDRAMNIOS

DEFINITION

Significantly increased risks that pregnancy will be complicated by: (1) maternal diabetes; (2) fetal anomaly; (3) PTL; (4) PROM; (5) MP

Acute

Late second or 3rd trimester; poor prognosis; 7:12 perinatal deaths

Chronic

Slow, early onset; better prognosis. Linked to maternal glucose intolerance, macrosomia, fetal anomalies

PHYSIOLOGY

Placenta then fetal urine excretion produces fluid. Fetal small bowel/diffusion through amnion/chorion absorbs. Most polyhydramnios is thought to be due to increased fetal urine production

DIAGNOSIS

Dye methods (inject/draw out dilution) 8% accurate

TIUV

AFI: Each quadrant, largest pocket measured in vertical axis. Sum of largest pockets in all four quadrants is AFI. 95th percent of amniotic fluid index during the 3rd trimester is 25 cm

(1) Observe weight gain
(2) Compare fundal height changes
(3) Palpate abdomen
(4) Perform ballottement for fetal parts
(5) Perform ultrasound – confirm polyhydramnios, detect multiple gestation, and obvious structural congenital malformation
    (a) BPD ventricle-to-hemisphere ratio
       HC vertebral column
    (b) Evaluate heart and chest cavity
    (c) Examine abdomen for ascites, abdominal masses, gastrointestinal atresia, abdominal wall masses, ompholocele or gastroschisis
    (d) Urinary system (kidneys, ureters, and bladder filling)
    (e) Evaluate skeletal system
    (f) Evaluate placenta
(6) Do 3-hr GTT
(7) Coombs' test (screen for irregular antibodies with indirect antiglobulin test)
(8) Amnio for karyotype analysis

ETIOLOGY

Idiopathic	60%
Diabetes mellitus	19%
Multiple gestation (Twin–Twin syndrome)	7.5%
Blood group incompatibility	5%
Congenital malformation	8.5%

MANAGEMENT

38 wks – PG/LS ratio
Bed rest
High-protein diet
Monitor serum proteins and use amnio to aspirate for SOB
Watch for CHF or IUGR
Sedation
No diuretics – little effect of TV of AF, may be harmful
Indomethacin (investigational) 50–100 mg p.o. t.i.d.–q.i.d.
Decreased AF production by decreasing fetal urine production
Dis: Premature closure of ductus arteriosis
            Fetal pulmonary hypertension
            Tricuspid insufficiency

Steps in delivery

(1)   Obtain fetal maturity studies – ultrasound, BPD, FL, head and abdominal circumferences, fetal lung maturity studies
(2)   Before induction – amnio p.r.n. to dec AF
(3)   Type and screen mother's blood
(4)   Baseline coagulation studies: platelets, CBC, fibrinogen
(5)   Controlled amniotomy with slow release of AF
(6)   Observe for placental separation
(7)   Observe for postpartum hemorrhage

ACUTE POLYHYDRAMNIOS (24–27 WKS)

(1)   Erythroblastosis fetalis ? Rx
(2)   Congenital malformations – term of pregnancy
(3)   If no cause – therapeutic amniocentesis
        500–1000 ml of AF
Tocolytics – MgS0$_4$ (3–5 g bolus over 30 min and then 2–5 g/hr [ ] 4–8 mg/dl), Brethine, NSAIDs (indomethacin 50–100 mg p.o. t.i.d.–q.i.d.)

Locate placenta

Hypoproteinemia – will develop; increase protein diet

Albumin IV p.r.n.

No diuretics

Antibiotics are contraindicated – can conceal early amnionitis

POST-DATE PREGNANCY

DEFINITION

Gestation 42 wks or greater

DIAGNOSIS

Correct assessment of gestational age
> Accuracy indirectly proportional to gestational age at time of assessment ("the earlier, the better")

Document
- (1) Regularity, length, date of last menses
- (2) Uterine size: 1st trimester/20 wks at umbilicus
- (3) Date of 1st fetal movement (quickening) 16–20 wks
- (4) Fetal heart rate detection (Doppler) 10–12 wks
- (5) U/S Dating: 1st trimester – CRL (error ± 3–5 days)
  - 2nd trimester – BPD, HC, FL (error ± 7–10 days)

Dating: – known LMP most accurate – *Naegele's Rule*
1st day of LMP – 3 months + 7 days = EDC
– known date of conception – using pregnancy wheel at 2 wks
– if LMP unsure – early U/S

COMPLICATIONS

- (1) Postmaturity – placenta maximally developed at 37 wks
  - – may decrease in surface area/function after 37 wks
  - – increased IUFD rates after 42 wks

- (2) Meconium – 25–30% of pregnancies ≥42 wks
  - – tends to be thicker secondary decreased AFV
  - – increased risk of meconium aspiration syndrome

- (3) Oligohydramnios – peak AFV @ 37 wks (~1000 cc)
  - – decreases to average 250 cc by 42 wks
  - – increased incidence of cord compression/acute hypoxia

- (4) Macrosomia – >4500 g, occurs in 2.5–10% at ≥42 wks
  - – increased risk of maternal/fetal trauma
  - – increased risk of shoulder dystocia

ANTEPARTUM MANAGEMENT

Cervical exam bi-weekly starting at 40 wks EGA
> *Favorable –* labor induction (oxytocin, prostin, arom, etc.)
> *Unfavorable –* surveillance vs cervical ripening (start at 41 wks)

SURVEILLANCE STRATEGY

(1)   *NST/AFI*   – reactive + AFI >5 = continue surveillance
                        – reactive + AFI <5 = biophysical profile or cervical ripening
                        – nonreactive and/or significant decelerations – cervical ripening

(2)   *Biophysical profile* (optional)
        >6 – continue surveillance

        ≤6 – cervical ripening

CERVICAL RIPENING

(1)   Prostaglandin E$_2$ gel 0.5 mg vs. vaginal suppository 2.5 mg q. 4 (or Cytotec 50 µg/25 µg)
        Check cervix before each dose:
        Favorable –   labor induction/augmentation
        Unfavorable – repeat prostaglandin application

(2)   Oxytocin – low-dose cervical ripening at l–2 mu/mtn

INTRAPARTUM MANAGEMENT

(1)   Continuous EFM   – persistent late decels/fetal intolerance of labor – Cesarean delivery
                                 – frequent variables – consider amnioinfusion

(2)   Suspect macrosomia   – avoid midpelvic operative delivery
                                 – EFW >5000 g – consider C-section

(3)   Determine presence of meconium
                – consider amnioinfusion
                – aggressive suctioning of infant on delivery of head (wall suction)

POST-DATE PREGNANCY

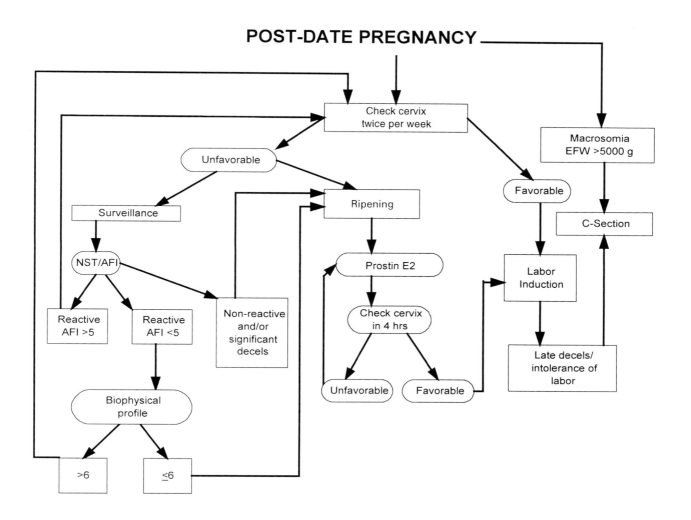

POSTPARTUM DEPRESSION

SYMPTOMS

Dysphoric mood

Loss of interest in usually pleasurable activities

Difficulty concentrating or making decisions

Psychomotor agitation or restriction

Fatigue

Changes in appetite or sleep

Recurrent thoughts of death/suicide

Feelings of worthlessness or guilt, especially failure at motherhood

Excessive anxiety over child's health

DOSE RANGES AND SIDE-EFFECT PROFILES OF ANTIDEPRESSANTS COMMONLY USED TO TREAT POSTPARTUM DEPRESSION

Drug gain	Therapeutic range (mg/day)	Side-effects[1]			
		Anticholinergic[2]	Orthostatic hypotension	Arrhythmia	Weight (>6 kg)
Tricyclics					
Amitriptyline (Elavil)	75–300	4+	4+	3+	4+
Desipramine (Norpramin)	75–300	1+	2+	2+	1+
Imipramine (Tofranil)	75–300	3+	4+	3+	3+
Nortriptyline (Pamelor)	40–200	1+	2+	2+	1+
SSRIs					
Fluoxetine (Prozac)	10–40	0	0	0	0
Paroxetine (Paxil)	20–50	0	0	0	0
Sertraline (Zoloft)	50–150	0	0	0	0

[1]0 = Absent or rare, 4+ = relatively common
[2]Dry mouth, blurred vision, urinary hesitancy, constipation, drowsiness

PRECOCIOUS PUBERTY

DEFINITION

Signs of secondary sexual maturation at an age 3 standard deviations below the mean for that population. In North America, this would be secondary sex characteristics before age 8, or menarche before age 9

EVALUATION

The two primary concerns of the parents are:
(1)   The social stigma ("different from peers")
(2)   Decreased height due to premature closure of epiphyseal growth centers

Subdivided into two classifications:
(1)   GnRH-dependent (complete, true, isosexual, central) – premature maturation of the hypothalamic–pituitary–ovarian axis. Usually the etiology is unknown. Is the most common
(2)   GnRH-independent (incomplete, pseudo, isosexual or heterosexual, peripheral) – independent of hypothalamic–pituitary control. The most common cause is an estrogen-secreting ovarian tumor (60% are granulosa cell tumors). McCune–Albright syndrome is a rare triad of café-au-lait spots, fibrous dysplasia, and cysts of the skull and long bones

DIFFERENTIAL DIAGNOSIS

75% of precocity in girls is idiopathic
Is very important to rule out a serious disease in the CNS, ovary, and adrenal gland

DIAGNOSTIC WORKUP

History and physical – must rule out life-threatening neoplasms of the ovary, adrenal, and CNS
Record height, weight and Tanner stages
Brain imaging studies (CT and/or MRI)
Serum estradiol, FSH, LH, TSH, triiodothyronine, thyroxine, prolactin, testosterone, DHEA or DHEAS, hCG
Bone age by hand-wrist films every 6 months to establish the rate of skeletal maturation
Abdominal ultrasound and/or CT to evaluate ovarian, uterine, or adrenal gland enlargement

LABORATORY FINDINGS

Laboratory findings in disorders producing precocious puberty

	Gonadal size	Basal FSH/LH	Estradiol or testosterone	DHEAS	GnRH response
Idiopathic	Increased	Increased	Increased	Increased	Pubertal
Cerebral	Increased	Increased	Increased	Increased	Pubertal
Gonadal	Unilater. incr.	Decreased	Increased	Increased	Flat
Albright	Increased	Decreased	Increased	Increased	Flat
Adrenal	Small	Decreased	Increased	Increased	Flat

From Speroff L, Glass RH, Kasc NG. *Clinical Gynecologic Endocrinology and Infertility*, 5th edn. Baltimore: Williams & Wilkins, 1994:375

TREATMENT

Depends on the cause, extent, and progression of precocious signs, and whether the cause can be removed operatively

Definitely treat:
(1)   Girls with menarche before age 8
(2)   Progressive thelarche and pubarche
(3)   Bone age over 2 years greater than their chronologic age

The drug of choice for GnRH-dependent precocious puberty is GnRH agonists
Maintain therapy until the median age of puberty. The drug of choice for McCune–Albright syndrome is testolactone. Both child and her family need intensive counseling

PREMATURE RUPTURE OF THE MEMBRANES (PROM)

DEFINITION

Premature rupture of membranes is defined as rupture of membranes prior to the onset of labor. It occurs in 6–20% of all pregnancies. Approximately 2/3 of patients with PROM before 37 wks are delivered within 4 days of rupture, and nearly 90% are delivered within one week

DIAGNOSIS

Making the correct diagnosis of PROM depends on a combination of history, physical examination and laboratory information

The patient's history alone is correct in over 90% of patients

Examination of the patient should be undertaken with an effort to avoid introducing infection. Digital intracervical examination in patients who are not in labor and for whom induction is not planned should be avoided, as such examinations add little needed information and probably increase the risk and complications of infection

Speculum examination should be undertaken to confirm the diagnosis, evaluate the general appearance of the cervix, take appropriate cultures, and rule out prolapse of the umbilical cord or fetal extremity

Confirmation of the diagnosis begins by identifying a pool of fluid in posterior vaginal fornix on speculum examination. This fluid may be tested using Nitrazine paper, or a drop may be allowed to dry on a slide, and when this is viewed under a microscope, ferning will be present if the fluid is from the amniotic cavity

Once the diagnosis of PROM is confirmed, four important questions must be answered before deciding on management:
(1)   The gestational age must be carefully assessed. Menstrual hx, prenatal exams and previous sonograms should be reviewed
(2)   The patient should be evaluated for the presence of chorioamnionitis. In cases of clinically apparent chorioamnionitis, signs will include fever, leukocytosis, maternal and fetal tachycardia, tender uterus and foul-smelling vaginal discharge
(3)   The patient should be evaluated for labor
(4)   The fetus should be evaluated for evidence of fetal distress

MANAGEMENT

Term

At 36 wks and beyond, the goal of management of PROM is delivery. In the absence of fetal distress or clinical infection, the patient should be observed for labor. There is no consensus of opinion as to when labor should be induced in a patient with PROM. However, patients should be allowed to go into labor spontaneously when possible. If labor has not begun within a reasonable time after rupture of membranes, induction with oxytocin may be acceptable

Pre-term

In pre-term pregnancies (less than 32 wks), conservative management is advocated, with intervention if signs of infection or fetal compromise are noted. Patients should be monitored carefully for evidence of infection. In asymptomatic patients, cultures for gonococci, chlamydia and group B streptococci are usually obtained. Prophylactic antibiotics are given until cultures are known to be negative. Also corticosteroids are considered for patients between 24–34 wks

In patients from 32–35 wks, fetal maturity assessment by collecting amniotic fluid vaginally, or by transabdominal amniocentesis, is carried out. If the 2:5 ratio or PG is positive, then delivery is usually advocated

Pre-viable or Pre-term PROM

A special set of problems must be considered in patients in whom membranes rupture very early in pregnancy (less than 25 wks). In these patients, there is relatively low likelihood (less than 25%) that a viable, gestational age will be achieved and the patient will deliver a surviving infant. Even in patients whose infants do survive, the vast majority deliver at very premature gestational ages, and many of the babies suffer significant short- and long-term morbidity

If the gestational age is early enough and the patient elects to terminate her pregnancy based on the low likelihood of a healthy baby, and some risk of maternal infectious sequela this is a reasonable option and should be discussed. If the patient elects to continue the pregnancy, expectant management is reasonable, with delivery indicated for chorioamnionitis, premature labor or other obstetric indications

PREMATURE RUPTURE OF THE MEMBRANES

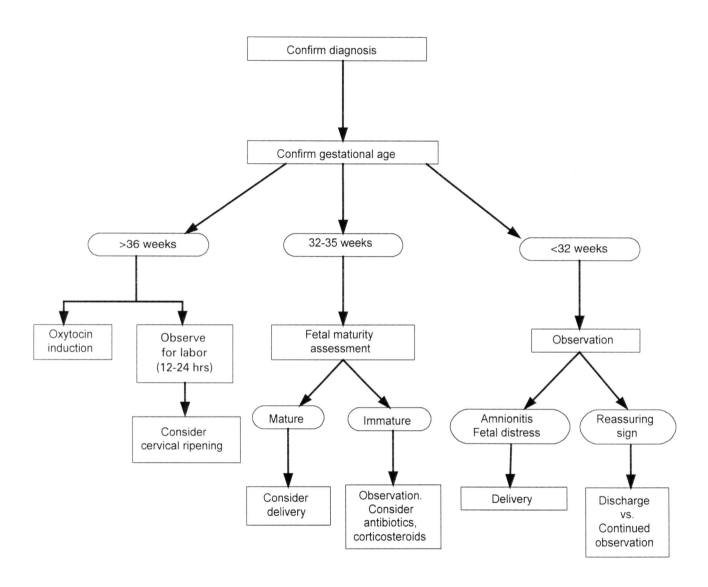

PREMENSTRUAL SYNDROME (PMS)

PMS may be defined as the cyclic recurrence, in the luteal phase of the menstrual cycle, of a combination of distressing physical, psychological, and/or behavioral changes of sufficient severity to result in deterioration of interpersonal relationships and/or interference with normal activities

The symptoms of PMS must appear during the luteal phase, which begins with ovulation, and diminish greatly or disappear with the onset of menstruation or shortly afterward. A woman who has symptoms throughout the cycle does not have PMS

DIAGNOSIS

The diagnosis of PMS is made with at least 2 months of documented ovulation and concurrent record-keeping of symptomatology disrupting lifestyle during the luteal phase. The symptom diary should be recorded daily throughout the month
Ask the patient to list three to five symptoms that bother her the most, and enter these on a daily symptom checklist for PMS. Have the patient track these symptoms for two menstrual cycles and bring the checklist back to you

PMS SYMPTOMS

Tension	Hypoglycemic episodes
Anxiety	Increased appetite
Mood swings	Headaches
Irritability	Sweet cravings
Depression	Weight gain
Confusion	Abdominal bloating
Crying	Breast tenderness
Forgetfulness	Swelling of extremities

Evaluation for PMS should include a history, physical exam and possibly laboratory studies. The history should elicit risk factors that correlate with PMS, sources of stress, medical or psychiatric problems, and physical or sexual abuse

The differential diagnosis of PMS includes molimina, situational stress disorders and chronic effective disorders

Molimina are the symptoms that women ordinarily experience premenstrually. They are the same as PMS symptoms, but are experienced to a lesser degree and allow women to continue their normal functions

Situational stress disorders result from major life changes such as divorce or a new job. The possibility of such stressors should be elicited in the history

The main feature distinguishing PMS from chorionic affective disorders is the follicular phase. Symptoms may be exacerbated premenstrually but these patients have some level of dysfunction throughout the entire cycle

The examiner should be looking for organic disease associated with PMS-type symptoms. These may include galactorrhea associated with hyperprolactinemia or pelvic pathology like ovarian cyst, endometriosis, leiomyomata or pelvic inflammatory disease associated with pelvic pain and distention. Most commonly the physical exam is normal

Some laboratory testing may be indicated. For those who complain of fatigue, a complete blood count, sedimentation rate, and chemistry panel are useful in detecting anemia or renal or liver abnormalities. Thyroid disease can cause fatigue and irritability, therefore thyroid function test may be ordered. Prolactin levels should be ordered on those with galactorrhea

NON-PHARMACOLOGIC TREATMENTS

Clinical experience indicates that patient education and support, stress reduction, a healthy diet, regular exercise and vitamin supplementations help many women both to understand and to feel more in control of their symptoms

DRUG THERAPIES

State-of-the-art treatment for PMS is with selective serotonin re-uptake inhibitors (SSRIs). When these don't work, an anxiolytic is usually next choice. Gonadotropin releasing hormone (GnRH) agonist may be used to suppress the menstrual cycle when symptoms are severe and respond to no other therapy

SSRIs

Start with half the recommended dosage for depression in order to reduce side-effects. If the patient tolerates this well, increase the dosage to 50 mg/d

Hold this dosage for one or two menstrual cycles to determine the degree of efficacy

ANXIOLYTICS

If an SSRI doesn't work, Alprazolam (Xanax) is usually the next choice

Start with 0.25 mg t.i.d., and increase as needed to control symptoms to a total of 1–1.25 mg/d

Buspirone HCl 10 mg (Buspar) p.o. t.i.d., taken throughout the cycle, may be effective

GnRH AGONIST

GnRH agonist can relieve the symptoms of PMS by producing a medical oophorectomy in patients for whom no other treatments work

PREMENSTRUAL SYNDROME

COPING WITH PMS

For women who suspect premenstrual syndrome (or who don't, but find that on some days things just don't go right!), there are several ways of coping that do not require a doctor's prescription

CHART YOUR SYMPTOMS

Finding out whether or not you are a victim of PMS can make you feel better. If you are a victim, knowing that you are not alone and understanding that the disorder is biochemical and not psychological can provide enormous relief

Talk about it

Talk about it with your husband, family, and even your employer – if necessary. You need their sympathy and support rather than having them tell you to 'pull yourself together' – which is exactly what someone with PMS cannot do. Your children also need to understand what PMS entails

Eat frequently and properly

Good nutrition, with reduced fats and increased complex carbohydrates, is important throughout your cycle, but even more so after ovulation, when it is especially vital to keep blood sugar on an even keel. The change in hormone levels then alters your biochemistry, making you more susceptible to low-blood-sugar reactions – such as irritability, migraines, panic, tears, angry outbursts. Never go for more than 4–5 hrs without food; a snack at bedtime may help, too

Exercise regularly

Half-hour aerobic workouts, in which you increase your pulse and work up a sweat, are good mood elevators. You should exercise three times a week all month

Cut down on salt

Since salt holds water, reducing salt intake should reduce bloating. In addition, do not add salt to your food. Cook with less and avoid high-sodium foods

Take vitamin supplements

The "B" vitamins – especially B_6 – are known to reduce bloating and have an antidepressant effect, and they seem to help control carbohydrate cravings. Suggested beginning daily dosage is a B-complex, containing 50 mg of B_6 daily, building up to 200–500 mg in a few months. Since B vitamins are water soluble, you will excrete what you don't need

Add bran to your diet

Some women become constipated during the premenstrual time and for the first few days of their period. Bran will bind water to itself and aid elimination. Be careful with alcohol. It may take only half your normal amount to make you merry!

Cut down on caffeine

This includes not only coffee but tea, cola, diet sodas, and chocolate as well. A group of substances (xanthines) in these encourages breast cysts: women who reduce intake of xanthines may find breasts are less tender during the premenstrual stage

Reduce stress if possible

Take things easy just before your period. If you're working, try to schedule important meetings and deadlines for another time of the month; at home, do not plan a dinner party or invite your cousin and her four kids for the weekend. Set aside some time to nap, listen to music, read, or go for a walk

Make love

Many women find that orgasm helps reduce pent-up tension. While masturbating may not be as good as sex with a loving partner, it also reduces pelvic congestion

The above are general recommendations for patients with symptoms of PMS. The actual PMS work-up can become quite complicated. SSRIs can be very helpful in this syndrome

PRE-OP LABS

The following labwork is required for ALL PATIENTS coming to the OR for surgery:

Age (years)	Men	Women
Under 40	None	Hgb or Hct
40–59	EKG BUN/glucose	EKG BUN/glucose Hgb or Hct
Over 60	EKG CXR BUN/glucose Hgb or Hct	EKG CXR BUN/glucose Hgb or Hct

SPECIAL NOTES

CXR is good for one year assuming no interval change in health

EKG is good for 6 months assuming no interval change in health

Blood work is good for 1 month assuming no interval change in health

These guidelines assume that the patient is otherwise in good health. Complicating factors (i.e. diabetes, hypertension, COPD) should obviously be considered for need to expand on these guidelines

PRE-TERM LABOR

DIAGNOSTIC CRITERIA FOR PRE-TERM LABOR

(1)   Gestational age between 20 and 37 wks
(2)   If the cervix is less than 2 cm dilated and less than 80% effaced, then cervical change is required to initiate tocolytic therapy
(3)   If the cervix is already >2 cm or >80% effaced, then therapy may be initiated when contractions occur with a frequency of four every 20 min or eight every 60 min, despite lateral bed rest and intravenous hydration

EVALUATION OF PRE-TERM LABOR

The initial evaluation of the patient with possible PTL has the following goals:
(1)   Confirm the diagnosis of PTL
(2)   Identify contraindications to tocolytic
(3)   Select the most appropriate tocolytic

A "STEP-BY-STEP" APPROACH

(1)   Lateral bed rest and intravenous fluids constitute care while a thorough obstetric and medical diagnosis is obtained
(2)   An external monitor assesses contractions and fetal well-being
(3)   A sterile speculum examination should be done to exclude PROM, and cultures vaginal Group B Streptococcus, cervical gonorrhea and chlamydia should be obtained
(4)   Ultrasound should be performed to confirm gestational age; to assess amniotic fluid volume; and fetal weight and position; to locate placenta and to rule out anomalies
(5)   Lab work should include a complete blood count and differential, urinalysis and culture, electrolytes and glucose and creatinine levels

CONTRAINDICATIONS TO TOCOLYSIS

Maternal	*Fetal*
Hypertension	Fetal demise or lethal anomaly
Cardiac disease	Amnionitis
Bleeding–abruption	Fetal distress
Hyperthyroidism	IUGR
	Gestational age >37 wks
	Birth weight >2500 g
	Cervical

177

CONTRAINDICATIONS FOR SPECIFIC TOCOLYTIC AGENTS

Beta-mimetic agents

Maternal cardiac rhythm disturbance or other cardiac disease

Poorly controlled diabetes, thyrotoxicosis or hypertension

Magnesium sulfate
  Hypocalcemia
  Myasthenia gravis
  Renal failure

Nifedipine
  Maternal liver disease

Indomethacin
  Asthma
  Coronary artery disease
  Gastrointestinal bleeding (active or past hx)
  Oligohydramnios
  Renal failure
  Suspected fetal cardiac or renal anomaly

POTENTIAL COMPLICATIONS OF TOCOLYTIC AGENTS

Beta-adrenergic agents
  Hyperglycemia
  Hypokalemia
  Hypotension
  Pulmonary edema
  Cardiac insufficiency
  Myocardial ischemia
  Maternal death

Magnesium sulfate
  Pulmonary edema
  Respiratory depression
  Cardiac arrest
  Maternal tetany
  Profound muscular paralysis
  Profound hypotension

Indomethacin
  Hepatitis
  Renal failure
  GI bleeding

Nifedipine
  Transient hypertension

TOCOLYTIC THERAPY WITH MAGNESIUM SULFATE

Procedure

(1) Loading
     4–6 g of magnesium sulfate (10% solution) IV slowly over 20-min period
(2) Maintenance
     Add 40 g of 50% magnesium sulfate solution to 920 cc D5W. Infuse at 2 g/hr (50 cc/hr). Infusion rate may be increased to 3 g/hr if uterine activity has not subsided in 30 min. Magnesium levels should be obtained before and after loading dose and at 2, 6 and 12 hrs during maintenance therapy. Therapeutic level 5–8 ng/l

(3)   Monitor
    (a)   Deep reflexes
    (b)   Respiration every 12 min
    (c)   Urinary output 25 cc or more per hour
    (d)   If deep reflexes are absent, discontinue immediately. Obtain magnesium sulfate level every 4 hrs

Calcium gluconate (1 g IV) is the antidote and must be available in labor rooms (10 ml 10% sol IV @ 3 min)

Magnesium sulfate infusion should be continued for a minimum of 10–12 hrs, after cessation of uterine activity. Strict intake and output charting should be maintained as magnesium sulfate does have cardiovascular side-effects

TERBUTALINE SULFATE THERAPY (Brethine)

Dosage and administration

Subcutaneous
(1)   Use a 25-gauge subcutaneous needle or 1-cc tuberculin syringe and obtain a 1-mg terbutaline sulfate
(2)   Administer terbutaline sulfate 0.25 sc initially and repeat every 30 min for a total of five doses (1.25 mg) as long as the maternal pulse rate is less than 120 BPM. **Notify physician if heart rate is over 120 BPM**
(3)   If premature labor has not been effectively arrested following initial therapy, terbutaline should be discontinued
(4)   If premature labor has been effectively arrested, begin maintenance subcutaneous dose as follows

Most patients
(1)   Terbutaline 0.25 mg sc every 6 hrs for 24 hrs
(2)   Maternal BP and pulse taken and recorded prior to each dose
(3)   Do not administer drug if maternal pulse is more than 120 BPM and notify physician
(4)   Should uterine activity persist during the maintenance therapy, administer a start dose (0.25 mg) and increase dose scheduled to 0.25 mg every 4 hrs for the remainder of 48-hr period as per physician's order. Should this regime become ineffective, therapy should be discontinued

Certain patients
Certain patients may be candidates for "treat and release" therapy. These will be patients with mild, poorly felt contractions without cervical changes who may be deemed to be in questionable or mild premature labor and whose contractions ceased within 6 hrs of initial therapy

Calcium channel blocking therapy (nifedipine)
Not recommended due to potential maternal hypotension, thus increased uteroplacental perfusion

Prostaglandin inhibitor therapy (sulindac or indomethacin)
Not recommended due to associated neonatal morbidity

Adjunctive therapy

Corticosteroids should be considered for the induction of fetal lung maturity. All women between 24 and 34 wks of pregnancy at risk for pre-term delivery are candidates for antenatal corticosteroid therapy

Betamethazone 12 mg IM in two doses 24 hrs apart *or*
Dexamethazone 5–6 mg q. 12 hrs for total of up to four doses

RESPIRATORY DISORDERS

RHINITIS OF PREGNANCY

Common causes of nasal congestion during pregnancy:

(1) **Allergic rhinitis** (most common)
Changes in cortisol levels
Rx: beclomethasone, topical Cromolyn, Sudafed (not if HTN)

(2) **Nasal polyposis**
Steroid burst will sometimes shrink polyps, but not recommended
Rx: sometimes has to be delayed until after pregnancy

(3) **Chronic sinusitis**
Rx: amoxicillin 500 mg t.i.d. x3 wks (E-mycin if allergic), Sudafed 60 mg b.i.d. or 30 mg q.i.d.

(4) **Rhinitis medicamentosa** (rebound rhinitis)
Occurs secondary to excessive use of over-the-counter decongestant nasal sprays
Rx: discontinue spray or drops. Give p.o. decongestants or intranasal corticosteroids

P.E. Oxymetazoline (vasoconstrictor – topical) to facilitate evaluation in patients who are not hypertensive

Character of mucous

(1) Copious clear secretions – allergic
(2) Yellowish/greenish discharge – infection

Epistaxis

(1) Intranasal saline spray 5–6x daily
(2) Eucerin/aloe b.i.d. in a.m. and p.m.
(3) Pinch nostrils and sit forward for 10 min

ASTHMA

(1) 4% of pregnancies
(2) ↑ PIH; hyperemesis; vaginal hemorrhage
(3) ↑ IUGR, PTD, LBW, neonatal hypoxia

Manage

(1) Baseline spirometry
(2) Peak expiratory flow daily – maintain 80% goal – Rx p.r.n.
(3) Early U/S, fetal kick count surveillance, NST/BPP p.r.n.
(4) EFM during exacerbation – maintain SaO_2 at 95% or >

Management of asthma exacerbations

(1) Rest, O_2, hydration, β_2-agonist Rx, EFM
(2) Hydrocortisone 100 mg IV to decrease risk of inflammatory mediated response 6–8 hrs later
(3) Oral steroids 1–2 wks pulsed course p.m. if inhaler not option
(4) Indentify asthma "triggers" – 75–80% have positive skin test
(5) Continue "allergy shots" in pregnancy if already been diagnosed
(6) Give annual influenza vaccine to pregnant patients if no egg allergy exists

(7)   Do not avoid physical activity
(8)   Cromolyn Na$^+$ inhaler regularly (mast cell stabilizer – prevents histamine release)
(9) β_2-agonist b.i.d.–q.i.d. inhaler
(10)   Oral prednisone/prednisolone p.r.n. (11β-ol-dehydrogenase metabolizes in placenta)
(11)   1-hr 50 g glucose CT at 27–30 wks secondary to increased risk of gestational DM
(12)   Severe exacerbation – inhaled nebulized β-agonists
       Terbutaline p.r.n.
       PTL – MgSO$_4$ prescription of choice
       Terbutaline requires increased dosing (ASA, NSAIDs, indomethacin, ibuprofen – 11% have
       hypersensitivities to these)

Management of labor

(1)   Continue regularly scheduled meds (except p.o. steroids)
(2)   If moderate to severe, check peak flow volume on admission then repeat every 12 hrs as
       needed
(3)   Maintain adequate hydration
(4)   Provide adequate analgesia
(5)   Avoid methergine and prostaglandin F2-alpha (Hemabate) – these are bronchoconstrictors.
       Use pitocin or prostaglandin E$_2$ as needed
(6)   Hydrocortisone 100 mg (or equivalent) IV every 8 hrs until 24 hrs postpartum
       Use #6 if patient has a history of p.o. steroid use at least 2 wks within previous 6 months or for
       those who have frequent exacerbations. This provides adrenal support and helps prevent
       exacerbations due to labor

Rh ISOIMMUNIZATION

D immunoglobulin administration to potentially susceptible candidates greatly reduces their chances of developing D isoimmunization and subsequent fetal morbidity/mortality of Rh hemolytic disease

PRENATAL TESTING

Determine maternal ABO and Rh type with prenatal profile at initial visit

Rh negative (not isoimmunized) women should have repeat D antibody determination at 28–29 wks EGA

> If negative, prophylactic D immunoglobulin (Rhogam)
> If positive, manage as D-sensitized

Presence of D-u (variant of D antigen) most often indicates maternal carriage of D-u antigen (considered Rh positive)

PROPHYLACTIC ADMINISTRATION (used only in unsensitized Rh women)

(1) Abortion (induced or spontaneous) and ectopic pregnancy
    (a) Up to 13 wks EGA – 50 µg D immunoglobulin
    (b) After 13 wks EGA – full dose (300 µg D immunoglobulin)
(2) Amniocentesis
    300 µg dose in 1st, 2nd or 3rd trimester. Follow with routine antepartum/postpartum prophylaxis. If delivery anticipated within 48 hrs, Rhogam may be held until postpartum
(3) Chorionic villus sampling
    50 µg dose D immunoglobulin
(4) Percutaneous Umbilical Cord Blood Sampling
    In D-negative women, analyze fetal blood. If D-positive, give 300 µg dose
(5) External version
    May precipitate fetal/maternal bleeding – 300 µg dose

SPECIAL SITUATIONS

(1) Antepartum placental hemorrhage
    (a) Kleihauer-Bettke to estimate volume of fetal–maternal transfusion
    (b) 300 µg dose protects against 30 ml fetal blood (15 ml fetal RBC)
    (c) May test 48–72 hrs after Rhogam dose for adequate treatment (excess D immunoglobulin = adequate treatment
(2) Postpartum/postabortal sterilization
    Controversial, but low risk of sensitization, probably precludes this group from treatment
(3) Administration of blood/blood products
    (a) Use of D-positive PRBC/platelets/granulocytes may cause sensitization
    (b) With D-positive PRBC – 300 µg per 15 ml PRBC (administered in six divided doses q. 12 hrs x72 hrs)
    (c) Platelets/granulocytes – single vial (300 µg) adequate

PREVENTION OF Rh ISOIMMUNIZATION

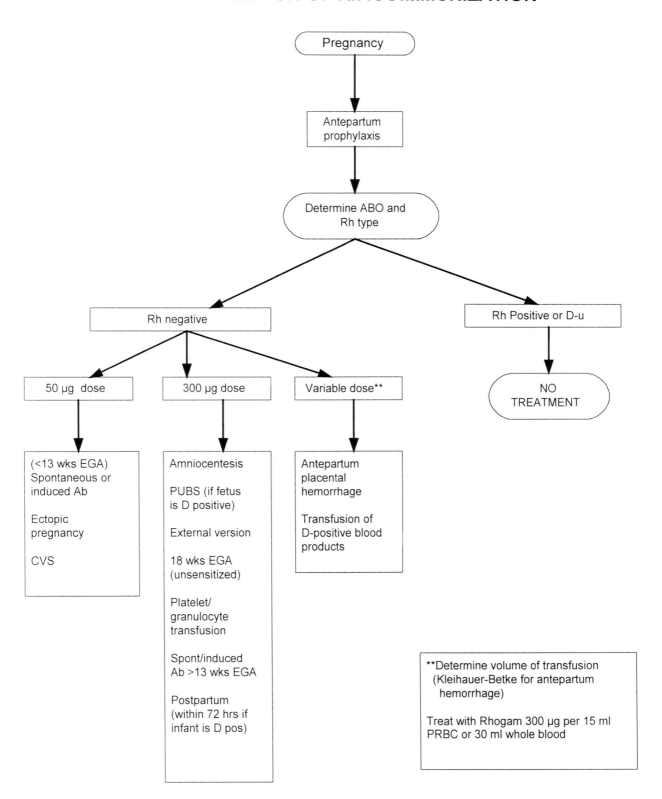

SCORING SYSTEMS

APGAR SCORING OF NEWBORNS

Sign	0 Points	1 Point	2 Points
Heart rate	Absent	Under 100	Over 100
Respiratory effort	Absent	Slow, irregular	Good, crying
Muscle tone	Limp	Some flexion	Active motion of extremities
Reflex irritability: response to catheter	No response	Grimace	Cough or sneeze, cry in nostril
Color	Blue–white	Body pink, extremities blue	Completely pink

BISHOP'S PELVIC SCORE

Features	0 Points	1 Point	2 Points	3 Points
Dilatation (cm)	0	1–2	3–4	5–6
Effacement (%)	0–30	40–50	60–79	80
Station	−3	−2	−1, 0	+1, +2
Consistency	Firm	Medium	Soft	—
Position	Posterior	Mid	Anterior	—

VAGINAL ATROPHY INDEX (VAI)

	1	2	3
Skin elast + turgor	Poor	Fair	Excellent
Pubic hair	Sparse	Normal	> Normal
Labia	Dry atrophy	Full	> Full
Introitus	<1 Fg br	1 Fg br	2 Fg br
Vaginal mucosa	Thin/friable	Sm	Rugated
Vaginal depth	Short	Normal	At least normal

VBAC SCORING SYSTEM (Flamm–Geiger)

<40 years of age	2 points
Vaginal delivery before and after their C-section	4 points
Vaginal birth after the first C-section	2 points
Vaginal birth before their Cesarean birth	1 point
No vaginal delivery	0 points
First C-section done for reason other than FTP	1 point
Cervix >75% on admission	2 points
Cervix 25–75% on admission	1 point
Cervix <25% on admission	0 points
Cervix dilated ≥4 cm on admission	1 point

0–2 points	49.1%	
3 points	59.9%	
4 points	66.7%	
5 points	77.0%	Likelihood of
6 points	88.6%	successful
7 points	92.6%	TOL
8–10 points	94.9%	

ZATUCHNI–ANDROS BREECH SCORE

	0 points	*1 point*	*2 points*
Parity	Primagrav.	Multip.	>
Gestational age	39 wks or >	38	37 or <
EFW	>8#	7–8#	<7#
Prev. breech	0	1	2 or >
Cx dil	2 cm	3 cm	4 cm or >
Station	−3 or higher	−2	−1 or lower

Total score of 5 or > indicates no difficulty in delivery of breech per vagina

SEPSIS

DEFINITIONS

Early sepsis ("warm shock")

Systemic response to infection (temp >38 °C, tachycardia, tachypnea, $PaCO_2$ <32 mmHg, WBC >12,000 or <4000 or >10% bands [i.e. left shift])

Late/severe sepsis ("cold shock")

Characterized by hypoperfusion, hypotension, organ dysfunction (peripheral cyanosis, cold extremities, lactic acidosis, oliguria, MS changes)

Septic shock

Sepsis accompanied by hypotension unresponsive to fluid resuscitation often requiring inotropic or vasopressor agents

Multiple organ system failure

Altered organ function such that homeostasis is not maintained without intervention

DIAGNOSIS

Clinical manifestations:

(1)   Cardiovascular
    (a)   Vasodilatation/increased vascular permeability – *hypotension*
    (b)   Myocardial depression – *cardiac dysfunction*
(2)   Pulmonary
    (a)   Vascular permeability/endothelial damage – *hypoxemia/ARDS*
(3)   Renal
    (a)   Hypotension/vasoconstriction – *oliguria*
    (b)   Prolonged cortical hypoxia – *ATN*
    (c)   Immune-mediated damage – *interstitial nephritis*
(4)   Hematologic
    (a)   Endotoxin activation of coagulation cascade – *DIC*
    (b)   Demargination/immune response – *leukocytosis*
(5)   Neurologic
    (a)   Decreased cerebral blood flow/hypoxia – *altered mental status*
(6)   Homeostatic
    (a)   Endotoxin/TNF effect on hypothalamus – *fever*

Laboratory investigation

(1)   CBC and platelets with differential
(2)   Electrolytes
(3)   Arterial blood gases
(4)   BUN/Cr
(5)   Urinalysis
(6)   Coagulation studies (PT/PTT, fibrinogen)
(7)   Serum lactate

(8) Cultures – blood, urine, other suspicious sites [endometrium, amniotic fluid, wound/episiotomy, sputum/drains]

(9) Radiologic studies – CXR +/– CT, MRI or abdominal X-ray

PRINCIPLES OF MANAGEMENT

Early (simple sepsis)

(1) Maintain adequate oxygenation (supplemental O_2)
(2) Maintain adequate circulating volume (IV fluids)
(3) Obtain appropriate laboratory data
(4) Initiate appropriate antibiotics (broad-spectrum)

Late (severe sepsis/shock)

(5) Transfer to Intensive Care (Swan–Ganz catheter)
(6) Surgical removal/drainage of abscess or infected tissue
(7) Tailor antibiotic coverage to culture results
(8) Institute inotropic/vasopressor agents

ANTIBIOTIC REGIMENS

(1) Ampicillin 2 g IV q. 6 hr + gentamicin (load: 2 mg/kg, maintenance: 1.5 mg/kg IV q. 8 hrs) + clindamycin 900 mg IV q. 8 hrs
(2) 3rd generation cephalosporin (cefotaxime 2.0 g IV q. 4 hrs or ceftriaxone 2.0 g IV q. 12 hrs or ceftazidime 2.0 g IV q. 8 hrs) + gentamicin (dose as in #1)
(3) Ticarcillin/clavulanate 6.2 g IV q. 6 hrs or piperacillin/tazobactam 6.75 g IV q. 6 hrs + gentamicin (dose as in #1)
(4) Cefoxitin 2.0 g IV q. 8 hrs + gentamicin (dose as in #1)

(PCN/cephalosporin allergic):
(5) Imipenem 500 mg IV q. 6 hrs
(6) Aztreonam 2.0 g IV q. 6 hrs + gentamicin (dose as in #1) + clindamycin 900 mg IV q. 8 hrs

INFECTION

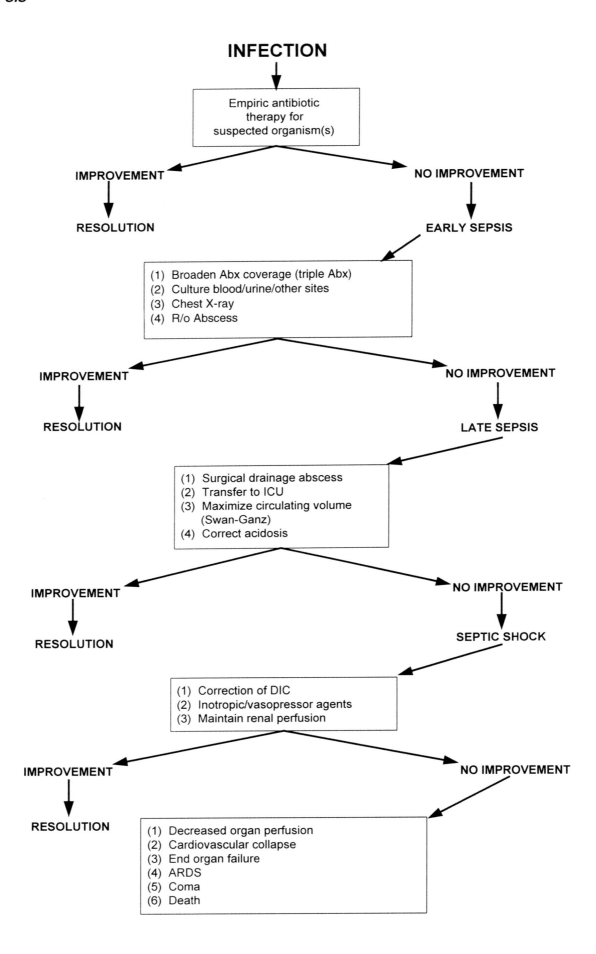

Empiric antibiotic therapy for suspected organism(s)

IMPROVEMENT   NO IMPROVEMENT

RESOLUTION   EARLY SEPSIS

(1) Broaden Abx coverage (triple Abx)
(2) Culture blood/urine/other sites
(3) Chest X-ray
(4) R/o Abscess

IMPROVEMENT   NO IMPROVEMENT

RESOLUTION   LATE SEPSIS

(1) Surgical drainage abscess
(2) Transfer to ICU
(3) Maximize circulating volume (Swan-Ganz)
(4) Correct acidosis

IMPROVEMENT   NO IMPROVEMENT

RESOLUTION   SEPTIC SHOCK

(1) Correction of DIC
(2) Inotropic/vasopressor agents
(3) Maintain renal perfusion

IMPROVEMENT   NO IMPROVEMENT

RESOLUTION

(1) Decreased organ perfusion
(2) Cardiovascular collapse
(3) End organ failure
(4) ARDS
(5) Coma
(6) Death

SEXUALLY TRANSMITTED DISEASES (STDs)

Chlamydia and Gonorrhea - see section on PID

Genital ulcers

Feature	Syphilis	Herpes	Chancroid	LGV	Granuloma inguinale
Incubation	2–4 wks	2–7 days	1–14 days	3d–6 wks	1–4 wks
Pain	Rare	Common	VERY tender	Varies	Uncommon
Lymph nodes	Firm, NT Bilat	Firm, NT Bilat	Tender, Sup Usu unilat	Tender Sup, loc	Pseudoadenopathy
Characteristics	*T. pallidum*	Resides dorsal root ganglia	*Hemophilus ducreyi*	*Chlamydia trachomatis*	*Calymmatobacterium granulomatis*
Diagnosis	Dark field microscopy	Cultures WBA	Gram Stain "School Fish" culture	Compliment fixation or culture Multiple fissures of perineum/ rectum	Find donovan bodies
Treatment	Penicillin B 2.4 million u	Acyclovir	Rocephin or erythromycin	Doxycycline	Tetracycline

THROMBOSIS

VIRCHOW'S TRIAD

Stasis, hypercoagulability, vessel wall abnormality

DIAGNOSIS OF DVT

Swelling of calf or thigh (unilateral)
Pain or tenderness
U/S (Venous Doppler)

DIAGNOSIS OF PE

Dyspnea and tachypnea

Pleuritic chest pain, hemoptysis, fever, panic, tachypnea, cyanosis, diaphoresis, friction rub, or changes in heart sounds
ABG (PaO_2) <85 mmHg
EKG — tachycardia, right axis shift
CXR — atelectasis?, pleural effusion?, increased diaphragm
Lung scan

TREATMENT

Heparin for 5–10 days. Monitor with APTT then subcutaneous heparin every 24 hrs in two divided doses for remainder of pregnancy. APTT levels should be obtained 6 hrs after subcutaneous dose

Heparin and warfarin Rx should overlap x4 days. (Warfarin can be started postpartum and thromboembolic episodes should be treated for at least 3 months)

Prophylactic heparin dosages

1st and 2nd trimester   5000–7500 units SQ b.i.d.
3rd trimester   10,000 units SQ b.i.d.
OR
Monthly U/S Doppler studies of lower extremities

Labor

D/c Heparin infusion 6 hrs prior to anticipated delivery. SQ Heparin may be withheld at onset of labor. Protamine reversal for APTT >1–1½ x control

Epidural contraindicated

Heparin infusion can be restarted when hemostasis is achieved (usually 2 hrs after delivery)

COMPLICATIONS

Hemorrhage 5–10%
Thrombocytopenia 3% (monitor platelets first 3 wks Rx – d/c if platelets <100,000)
Osteoporosis – (supplemental Vit D rec for long-term Rx)
Increased liver enzymes

REVERSE

Protamine sulfate 1 mg/100 units of heparin
(Do not exceed 100 mg)

THROMBOSIS

HEPARIN DOSING GUIDELINES

(1)   Obtain patient's weight in kg = _____

(2)   Calculate bolus dose 80 units/kg = _____units IV

(3)   Standard heparin infusion is 10,000 units of heparin in 250 ml D5W

      IV heparin maintenance dose 15–25 U/kg/hr = _____ units/hr

(4)   Warfarin _____ mg. Begin day 1–3 heparin therapy (if postpartum)

Weight	Loading dose	Maintenance dose
≤149 lb (≤70 kg)	5,000 units	1,000 units/hr (25 ml/hr)
150–200 lb (71–90 kg)	7,500 units	1,400 units/hr (35 ml/hr)
≥201 lb (≥91 kg)	10,000 units	1,800 units/hr (45 ml/hr)

Dose adjustments

APTT	Rate change (ml/hour)	Dose change
<36 sec	+5	+200 U, 5,000 U bolus
36–44 sec	+3	+120 U, no bolus
45–73 sec	0	none
74–90 sec	−3	−120 U, stop heparin x1 hr
>90 sec	−3	−120 U, stop heparin x1 hr

APTT, Activated partial thromboplastin time

TRAUMA

INITIAL BLOOD STUDIES

Complete blood cell count with platelets

DIC (disseminated intravascular coagulation) screen (fibrinogen, platelets, prothrombin time, partial thromboplastin time, fibrin-split products)

Biochemistries

Amylase

Kleihauer–Betke test (particularly if Rho(D)-negative)

Type and cross-match

ANATOMIC AND PHYSIOLOGIC CHANGES RELEVANT TO TRAUMA MANAGEMENT DURING PREGNANCY

Anatomic/physiologic change	Relevance to trauma anagement	Implication/action
Increased maternal blood volume	Increases by up to 50% in the 3rd trimester	Blood loss may be underestimated
Increased RBC mass	RBC mass increases to a lesser degree than total plasma volume, resulting in decreased hematocrit	Hematocrit as low as 30–32% may be physiologic
Decreased blood pressure	Blood pressure decreases by 10–15% mmHg, particularly in the midtrimester	Must be taken into consideration when evaluating for hypovolemia/hemorrhagic shock
Increased pulse rate	Pulse rate increases by 5–10 beats/min during pregnancy	Same as above
Decreased gastrointestinal motility	Gastric emptying time is prolonged, increasing risk for aspiration	Consider use of nasogastric tubes when aspiration is a risk
Cephalad displacement of intra-abdominal contents	Small bowel is compressed within the upper abdomen in latter pregnancy	Penetrating trauma to the upper abdomen is likely to cause complex intestinal injuries
Respiratory rate increases	pCO_2 is normally 32 mmHg; pCO_2 in the 'normal' range (40–42 mmHg) may indicate impending respiratory failure	
Bladder is displaced superiorly into the abdomen after 12 weeks' gestation	Bladder is subject to blunt or penetrating injury with lower abdominal trauma	Suspect bladder injury in traumatic events to the lower abdomen

TRAUMA

ESTIMATION OF BLOOD LOSS BASED ON CLINICAL VARIABLES

	Class I	Class II	Class III	Class IV
Blood loss (ml)	Up to 750	750–1500	1500–2000	≥2000
Blood loss (% BV)	Up to 15%	15–30%	30–40%	≥40%
Pulse rate	<100	>100	>120	≥140
Blood pressure	Normal	Normal	Decreased	Decreased
Pulse pressure (mmHg)	Normal or increased	Decreased	Decreased	Decreased
Capillary blanch test	Normal	Positive	Positive	Positive
Respiratory rate (min)	14–20	20–30	30–40	>35
Urine output (ml/hr)	≥30	20–29	5–15	Negligible
CNS/mental status	Slightly anxious	Mildly anxious	Anxious and confused	Confused/lethargic
Fluid replacement (3:1 rule)	Crystalloid	Crystalloid	Crystalloid + blood	Crystalloid + blood

INTERPRETATION OF DIAGNOSTIC PERITONEAL LAVAGE (POSITIVE)

Free aspiration of blood (>10 ml)

Grossly bloody lavage fluid

RBC count >100,000/mm^3

WBC count >500/mm^3

Amylase >175

INDICATIONS FOR DIAGNOSTIC PERITONEAL LAVAGE DURING PREGNANCY

Abdominal signs or symptoms suggesting intraperitoneal hemorrhage

Unexplained shock

Altered mental status

Major thoracic injuries

Multiple major orthopedic injuries (including pelvic fracture)

TRAUMA IN PREGNANCY

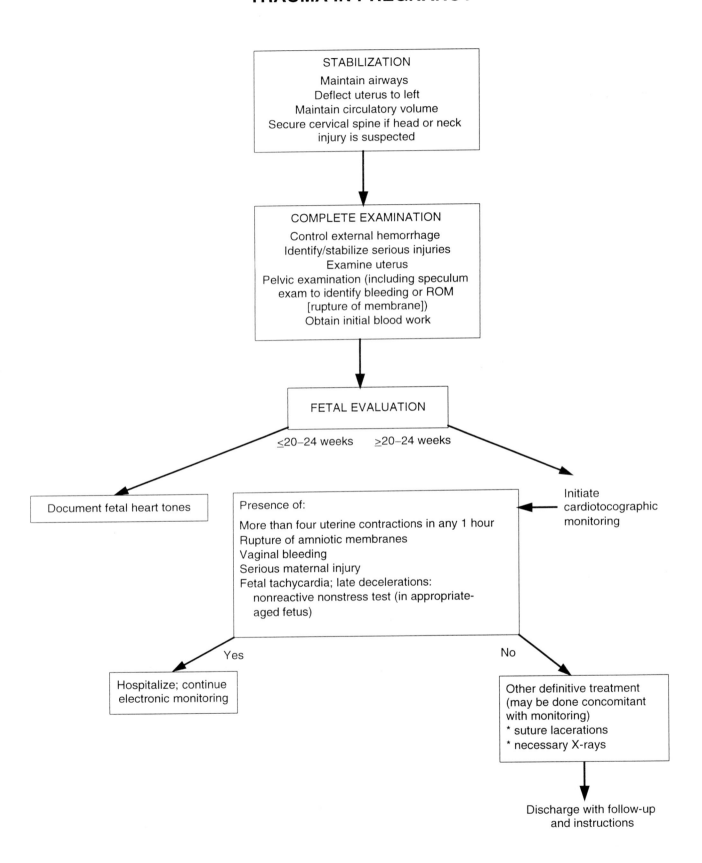

STABILIZATION

Maintain airways
Deflect uterus to left
Maintain circulatory volume
Secure cervical spine if head or neck
injury is suspected

COMPLETE EXAMINATION

Control external hemorrhage
Identify/stabilize serious injuries
Examine uterus
Pelvic examination (including speculum
exam to identify bleeding or ROM
[rupture of membrane])
Obtain initial blood work

FETAL EVALUATION

≤20–24 weeks   ≥20–24 weeks

Document fetal heart tones

Initiate
cardiotocographic
monitoring

Presence of:

More than four uterine contractions in any 1 hour
Rupture of amniotic membranes
Vaginal bleeding
Serious maternal injury
Fetal tachycardia; late decelerations:
   nonreactive nonstress test (in appropriate-
   aged fetus)

Yes   No

Hospitalize; continue
electronic monitoring

Other definitive treatment
(may be done concomitant
with monitoring)
* suture lacerations
* necessary X-rays

Discharge with follow-up
and instructions

TROPHOBLASTIC DISEASE

DEFINITION

Constitutes a spectrum of tumors and tumor-like conditions characterized by a proliferation of pregnancy-associated trophoblastic tissue of progressive malignant potential

LESIONS INCLUDE:

(1)   Hydatidiform mole
    (a)   complete
    (b)   partial
(2)   Invasive mole (chorioadenoma destruens)
(3)   Frankly malignant choriocarcinoma
(4)   Placenta site tumors

The important reason for the correct recognition of the true moles is that they are the most common precursors of choriocarcinoma

HYDATIDIFORM MOLE

Complete

Is 46XX or XY coming from father 90% of the time

No evidence of fetal tissue

All the chorionic villi are involved and markedly edematous

Fetal vessels are absent

10–30% progress to persistent trophoblastic disease

2–3% will develop choriocarcinoma

Partial mole

Usually triploid 69 XXY, XYY

hCG titers are seldom as elevated as in complete mole

A fetus is usually present at some point

Are composed of a mixture of normal-sized chorionic villi mixed with large hydropic ones

Most persistent gestational trophoblastic disease after a partial mole is confined to the uterus, with choriocarcinoma exceedingly rare

The clinical follow-up is the same

Invasive mole

Is defined as a mole that penetrates and may even perforate the uterine wall

The tumor is locally destructive and may invade parametrial tissue or blood vessels

Hydropic villi may embolize to distant sites as lungs and brain, but do not grow in these organs as true metastasis

It is associated with persistent elevated hCG

Responds well to chemotherapy

Choriocarcinoma

Is an epithelial malignancy of trophoblastic cells derived from any form of previously normal or abnormal pregnancy

Most cases arise in the uterus, ectopic pregnancies provide extrauterine sites of origin

Is rapidly invasive, widely metastasizing malignancy, but once identified responds well to chemotherapy

Arise in 1/20,000–30,000 pregnancies in USA

50% arise in hydatidiform moles

25% previous abortion

25% normal pregnancies

Classically the uterus choriocarcinoma does not produce a large, bulky mass

It becomes manifest only by irregular spotting of bloody, brown, sometimes foul-smelling fluid

Widespread metastases are characteristic of these tumors. Lungs 50%; vagina 30–40%; followed by brain, liver and kidney

Placenta site tumors

Is a rare tumor characterized by the presence of proliferating trophoblastic tissue deeply invading the myometrium and is composed largely of an intermediate trophoblast

There is a low level of hCG

The tumors are locally invasive, but many are self-limited and subject to cure by curettage

About 10% result in disseminated metastasis and death

Are not sensitive to chemotherapy

Hysterectomy is the treatment of choice

MANAGEMENT

In patients in whom hydatidiform mole is suspected prior to evacuation, the following studies should be done:
(1)   CBC with platelets
(2)   Clotting function studies
(3)   Renal and liver functioning studies
(4)   Blood type and antibody screen
(5)   Blood available
(6)   β-hCG level
(7)   Chest X-ray

If the patient desires surgical sterilization, a hysterectomy may be performed with the mole *in situ*. The ovaries may be preserved at the time of surgery. Hysterectomy eliminates the risk associated with local invasion, but it doesn't prevent distant spread

Suction curettage is the preferred method of evacuation in patients who desire to preserve fertility
Intravenous oxytocin begun after the cervix is dilated
After completion of suction curettage, gentle sharp curettage may be performed

PROPHYLACTIC CHEMOTHERAPY

It is controversial

May be particularly useful in the management of high-risk molar pregnancy, especially when hormonal follow-up is unavailable or unreliable

Patients at high risk

(1)   hCG level >100,000
(2)   Excessive uterine enlargement
(3)   Theca lutein cyst >6 cm
(4)   Age more than 40

Follow-up

After molar evacuation, patient should be followed-up by weekly determinations of β-hCG levels until these are normal for 3 consecutive weeks and then by monthly determinations until levels are normal for 6 consecutive months

The β-hCG level should become negative by 8–12 weeks
Contraception is recommended for at least 6 months to 1 year after remission

Patients with a prior partial or complete molar gestation have 10-fold increased risk (1–20% incidence) of a second mole in subsequent pregnancies

If β-hCG values rise or plateau over more than 2 weeks, immediate work-up and treatment for malignant post-molar GTD is indicated

Classification of GTD

Benign GTD
(1)   Complete
(2)   Incomplete

Malignant GTD
(1)   Non-metastatic GTD – virtually all patients can be cured using single-agent chemotherapy
(2)   Metastatic GTD
(a)   Good prognosis – low risk, absence of risk factor. These are likely to respond to single-agent chemotherapy
(b)   Poor prognosis (high risk)
(i)   Duration >4 months
(ii)   Pretherapy level of β-hCG in serum >40,000 mIU/ml
(iii)   Brain or liver metastasis
(iv)   GTD after term gestation
(v)   Prior failed therapy

Prophylactic chemotherapy can be given to high-risk patients

TUBO-OVARIAN ABSCESS (TOA)

MANAGEMENT OF THE PATIENT WITH A PELVIC ABSCESS

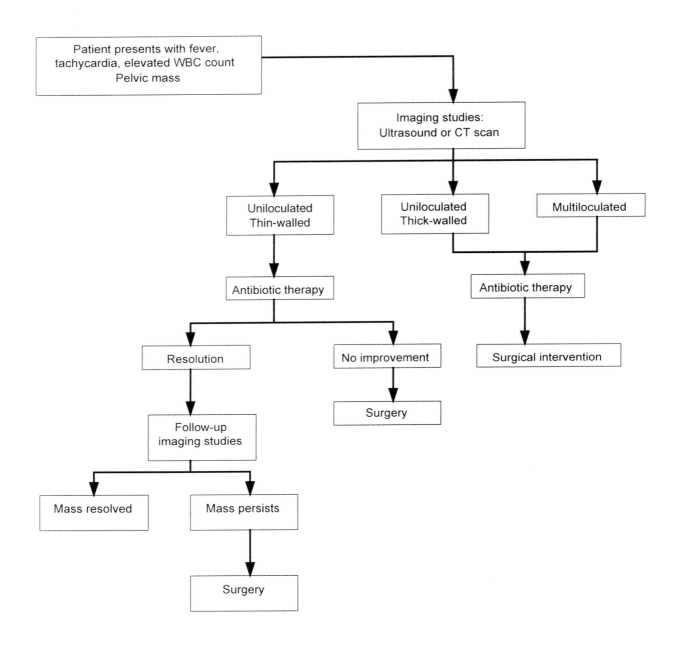

TUBO-OVARIAN ABSCESS (TOA)

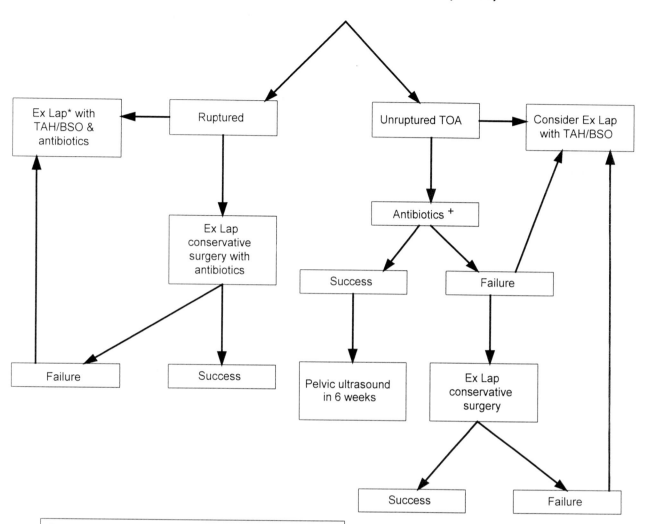

+**CDC Inpatient Treatment Regimens**

Regimen A: Cefoxitin, 2 g IV q. 6 hrs or cefotetan,
2 g IV q. 12 hrs, plus doxycycline,
100 mg IV/p.o. q. 12 hrs

Regimen B: Clindamycin, 900 mg IV q. 8 hrs plus
gentamicin, loading dose 2 mg/kg
followed by maintenance dose of
1.5 mg/kg q. 8 hrs

*Ex Lap, exploratory laparotomy

TWINS

INCIDENCE

1 : 95 in US

WEIGHT GAIN

(1) 24 lb by 24 weeks' gestation
(2) 40–70 lb total okay

VISITS

(1) Biweekly until 20 weeks and then weekly after 32 weeks
(2) House calls p.r.n.
(3) Cervical checks (?) p.r.n. U/S or digital
(4) U/S at 18 weeks
(5) U/S + NST from 28–30 weeks' gestation
(6) BPP if NSTs are non-reactive and equivocal or U/S demonstrates discordant growth

DECREASE OF PHYSICAL ACTIVITY AFTER 28 WEEKS

(1) If IUGR of one or both twins is suspected, patient to be placed on strict bed rest at home or in hospital to monitor each twin's growth closely by serial ultrasound measurements of BPB, head circumference, and femur length
(2) Examine for twin–twin syndrome, etc.

INTRAPARTUM MANAGEMENT TO INCLUDE:

(1) Fetal monitoring throughout labor
(2) U/S needs to be in labor and delivery room in the event that version is required for a second twin
(3) Epidural anesthesia is preferred to facilitate manipulation of the second twin in addition to relieving pain
(4) OR staff would be required to be on stat back-up secondary to the anticipated vaginal delivery of second twin which may need to be reversed at a moment's notice
(5) C-section might be required if advanced labor with premature twin gestations is noted between 26–34 weeks' gestation
(6) C-section would be strongly considered if the first twin's presentation is shoulder, transverse, or breech
(7) If the second twin is breech and the first twin is vertex, the first twin could be delivered if there are no other complications followed by external version, internal version, partial breech extraction with piper forceps of the second twin under general anesthesia using halothane for uterine relaxation p.r.n. (C-section may be required for the delivery of the second twin in these cases)

TWIN TYPES

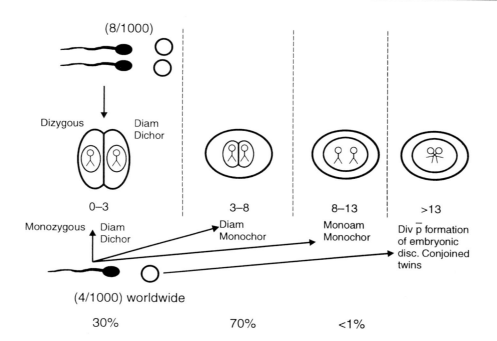

(8/1000)

Dizygous · Diam Dichor

0–3

Monozygous · Diam Dichor → Diam Monochor → Monoam Monochor · Div p̄ formation of embryonic disc. Conjoined twins

3–8

8–13

>13

(4/1000) worldwide

30%

70%

<1%

TWO-VESSEL CORD

ETIOLOGY

(1) Fails to form (aplasia or agenesis)
(2) Involutes after forming (atrophy)

20% SUA have associated abnormalities

ASSOCIATED WITH VARIETY OF FETAL ABNORMALITIES

Trisomy 18 ⎫
           ⎬ increased rate 10% (0.5–1% normally)
Trisomy 13 ⎭

When one artery is missing the *most common* anomaly is one kidney missing

(1) Increased rate IUGR   ⎫
                                              ⎬ x2 increase
(2) Increased rate PTL and preterm birth   ⎭
(3) Increased rate of *spontaneous abortion*
(4) *Frequently* observed in *multiple pregnancies*
(5) *Seen more frequently* in conjunction with fetal malformations

CNS anomalies
Cardiac defects
GI defects
     Esophageal atresia   ⎫
     Tracheoesophageal fistula   ⎬ x5 increase
     Anorectal atresia   ⎭
Multicystic dysplastic kidneys
Limb reduction defects

Velamentous cord insertions   }   increased 2.7 (1% gen OB pts)

SONOGRAPHIC DIAGNOSIS

Many obstetricians have never noticed an umbilical cord with a single umbilical artery *in utero*

(1) Almost impossible to detect a single umbilical artery without a 5-MHz transducer and challenging even with a 5-MHz scan head
(2) Not all imaging studies include a careful look at the umbilical cord vasculature
(3) May become atretic after the original study is done

Once the fetus is determined to have just one umbilical artery:

(1) Assess growth and fluid volume
(2) See if determination can be made of where the cord enters the placenta
(3) Offer amniocentesis
(4) Provide PTL information and cautions
(5) NSTs >32 wks (2 degrees to increased rate stillbirth)

EVALUATION/MANAGEMENT OF PREGNANCY
WITH A TWO-VESSEL CORD

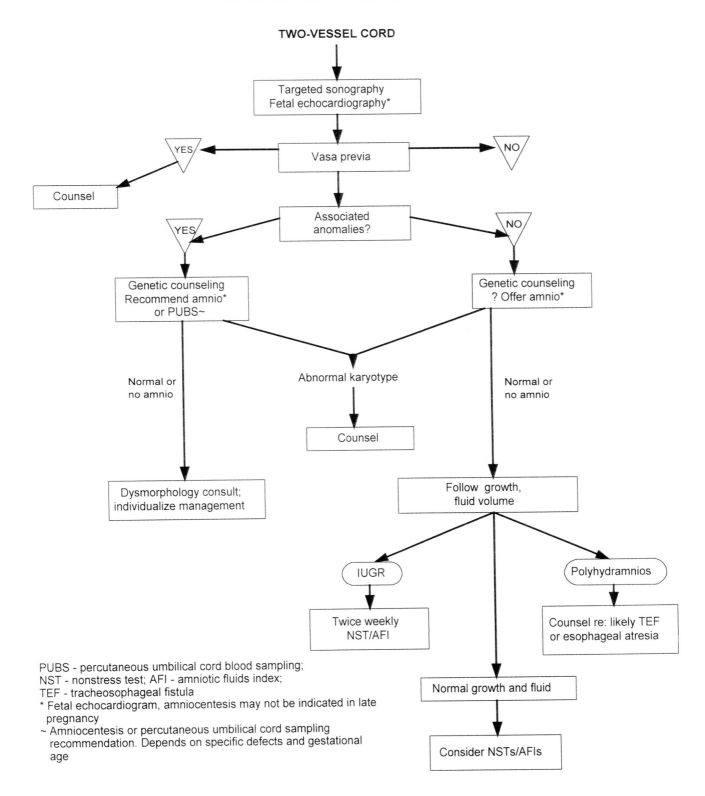

PUBS - percutaneous umbilical cord blood sampling;
NST - nonstress test; AFI - amniotic fluids index;
TEF - tracheosophageal fistula
* Fetal echocardiogram, amniocentesis may not be indicated in late
  pregnancy
~ Amniocentesis or percutaneous umbilical cord sampling
  recommendation. Depends on specific defects and gestational
  age

UMBILICAL CORD BLOOD GAS ANALYSIS

FETAL/NEWBORN ACIDEMIA (3 TYPES)

(1)   Respiratory – pCO_2 high, HCO_3 normal
(2)   Metabolic   – pCO_2 normal, HCO_3 low
(3)   Mixed   – pCO_2 high, HCO_3 low
Umbilical artery pH and blood gas – adjunct to Apgar scores

TECHNIQUE

(1)   10–20 cm cord segment clamped on either end
(2)   Perform immediately after delivery
(3)   Aspirate umbilical *artery*
(4)   Sample may be obtained from chorionic surface of placenta
      (arteries cross *over* veins)
(5)   1–2 cc sample aspirated into heparinized syringe
(6)   Residual air bubble expelled
(7)   Cord segment sample stable for 1 hour at room temp
'Normal' umbilical artery pH = 7.27 (mean)
±2 standard deviations = 7.15–7.39

Pathologic fetal acidemia

Traditional threshold <7.20

Realistic threshold (i.e. pH associated with adverse neonatal sequelae, neurologic dysfunction/death) <7.0

Birth asphyxia/hypoxia = low Apgars (0–3 at 5 minutes) + pH <7

PROTOCOL

(1)   Doubly clamp cord segment (10–20 cm) immediately after birth in all deliveries and place on table

(2)   pH and acid–base determinations indicated for:
      – prematurity
      – meconium (requiring tracheal visualization, suctioning and/or intubation)
      – nuchal cord
      – low Apgar scores (<7 at 5 minutes)
      – abnormal antepartum fetal heart tracing
      – any serious problem with delivery or neonate's condition

(3)   If unable to obtain cord specimen, aspirate artery on chorionic surface of placenta

(4)   Discard cord segment if 5 minute Apgar score satisfactory and newbom stable/vigorous

UTERINE BLEEDING

MANAGEMENT IN ADOLESCENTS

Within the first year of menarche approximately 55% of cycles are anovulatory. The hypothalamic–pituitary–ovarian axis takes time to mature and to develop its finely tuned feedback system. Up to a third of adolescents still have anovulatory cycles in the fifth year of menarche

POSSIBLE CAUSES OF MENORRHAGIA

Anovulation

Hypothalamic dysfunction
Polycystic ovary disease

Pregnancy-related conditions

Threatened or spontaneous abortion
Retained products of conception after elective abortion

Primary coagulation disorders

Systemic diseases

Diabetes mellitus
Hepatic dysfunction
Renal dysfunction
Thyroid dysfunction

Trauma

Accidental injury
Coital trauma
Sexual abuse

Lower reproductive tract infections

Chlamydia
Pelvic inflammatory disease

Neoplasms

Endometrial hyperplasia
Hormonally active ovarian tumors
Leiomyoma
Vaginal tumors

Iatrogenic causes

Exogenous hormone use
Ingestion of medications containing estrogenic activity

OFFICE EVALUATION OF BLEEDING

(1)   A complete menstrual history, including the following:
- (a)   Date of menarche
- (b)   Frequency and regularity of menstrual cycles
- (c)   Date of onset of most recent period or bleeding episode
- (d)   An estimate of the number of pads used per day
- (e)   Whether the patient has cramps or pain, clotting, or symptoms of syncope or nausea with menses

(2)   Ask about history of excessive bleeding after surgical or dental procedures and any family history of endocrine or coagulation disorders

(3)   Ask the patient whether she has been sexually active; whether she has used any method of contraception; and whether she feels there is any possibility of pregnancy. This interview must be done in privacy, after an explanation to mother and daughter of the importance of confidentiality in the relationship of a physician to an adolescent

LABORATORY TESTS

Complete blood counts
Platelet counts
Pregnancy test
Thyroid function test

For severe bleeding
    bleeding time
    partial thromboplastin time
    prothrombin time
    serial hemoglobin and hematocrit
    type and screen

THERAPY

A patient who is mildly anemic will benefit from hormonal management
(1)   Combination low-dose oral contraceptive; then re-evaluate after 3–6 cycles to decide whether to continue this regimen
(2)   An alternative is: medroxyprogesterone 5 to 10 mg/day for 10–14 days

Patients with heavy bleeding, but who are stable, will require higher-dose hormonal therapy
(1)   Monophasic OC (Ovral) two pills until stop bleeding – then one daily

ACUTE BLEEDING: EMERGENCY MANAGEMENT

(1)   Either conjugated estrogens 25–40 mg IV every 4–6 hrs or oral estrogen 2.5 mg every 6 hrs, will be effective x 24 hrs
(2)   If not, a D&C is indicated
(3)   The failure of hormonal management suggests that a local cause of bleeding is more likely
(4)   If IV or oral estrogen controls the bleeding successfully, oral progestin therapy must be added and continued for several days to stabilize the endometrium. This therapy can be accomplished by switching to a combination oral contraceptive
(5)   Remember that up to 19% of patients hospitalized with heavy uterine bleeding had an underlying coagulation disorder

UTERINE INVERSION

MANAGEMENT OF ACUTE PUERPERAL UTERINE INVERSION

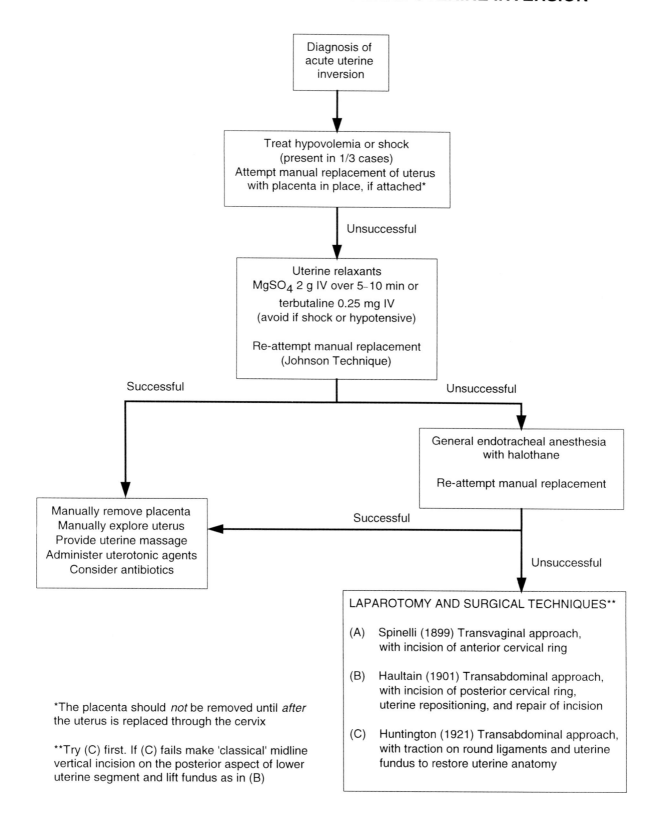

Diagnosis of acute uterine inversion

Treat hypovolemia or shock
(present in 1/3 cases)
Attempt manual replacement of uterus
with placenta in place, if attached*

Unsuccessful

Uterine relaxants
$MgSO_4$ 2 g IV over 5–10 min or
terbutaline 0.25 mg IV
(avoid if shock or hypotensive)

Re-attempt manual replacement
(Johnson Technique)

Successful   Unsuccessful

General endotracheal anesthesia
with halothane

Re-attempt manual replacement

Manually remove placenta
Manually explore uterus   Successful
Provide uterine massage
Administer uterotonic agents
Consider antibiotics

Unsuccessful

LAPAROTOMY AND SURGICAL TECHNIQUES**

(A)   Spinelli (1899) Transvaginal approach,
      with incision of anterior cervical ring

(B)   Haultain (1901) Transabdominal approach,
      with incision of posterior cervical ring,
      uterine repositioning, and repair of incision

(C)   Huntington (1921) Transabdominal approach,
      with traction on round ligaments and uterine
      fundus to restore uterine anatomy

*The placenta should *not* be removed until *after* the uterus is replaced through the cervix

**Try (C) first. If (C) fails make 'classical' midline vertical incision on the posterior aspect of lower uterine segment and lift fundus as in (B)

UTERINE RUPTURE

Uterine rupture: 1 in 1148–2250

TYPES OF UTERINE RUPTURE

(1)   Complete
(2)   Incomplete

CLASSIC SIGNS

(1)   Vaginal hemorrhage
(2)   Shock
(3)   Cessation of labor
(4)   Recession of the presenting part

78% of patients with uterine rupture have evidence of fetal distress prior to onset of bleeding or pain. Fetal distress and loss of uterine contractions in patients with a history of previous uterine scar puts diagnosis of uterine rupture high on differential diagnosis

Examine uterus directly after delivery of placenta and before uterus contracts

MANAGEMENT

(1)   Silent dehiscence
    (a)   SVD – observation with expectation of spontaneous healing – plan R. C/S
    (b)   R. C/S – repair at time of R/CS

(2)   Symptomatic rupture – emergency hysterectomy

    Causes of emergency hysterectomy:
    (a)   Atony (43%)
    (b)   Placenta accreta (30%)
    (c)   Uterine rupture (13%)
    (d)   Extension of low transverse scar (10%)

(3)   Complete rupture
    (a)   Intact uterus – 13.5% maternal mortality
    (b)   Scarred uterus – 0% maternal mortality
    (c)   Intact uterus – 76% fetal mortality
    (d)   Scarred uterus – 32% fetal mortality

SUSPECT UTERINE RUPTURE

HISTORY:

Previous uterine surgery (C/S, hysterotomy, myomectomy, metroplasty)
Trauma (MVA, Ab, Exc fundal pressure, MFR, PPD&C, manual removal of placenta, penetrating wounds, uterine manipulations)
Inappropriate use of Pitocin
Multiparity
Fetal factors (macrosomia, malposition, anomalies)
Uterine anomalies (acquired – gest neoplastic dis, adenomyosis, cocaine abuse, ART reprod techniques)
Overdistension (hydramnios, multiple pregnancies)

SIGNS AND SYMPTOMS:

Maternal anxiety
Fetal distress/demise
Pain not assoc w/ contractions
Vaginal bleeding
Vascular instability & shock
Cessation of labor
Recession of presenting part
Easily palpable fetal parts @ abdomen
Point tenderness of uterus
U/S evidence of rupture
Extrusion of uterine contents
Decompression of IUPC
Signs of peritoneal irritation (chest pain/shoulder pain)
Firmly contracted uterus and cardiovascular collapse w/ or w/o heavy vaginal bleeding

Silent dehiscence

Symptomatic

Found at time of SVD or VBAC

Found at time of C-section

Emergency hysterectomy

Observe

Repair

Compress aorta to save time p.r.n.

Plan R. C/S at next pregnancy

Consider saving uterus only in rare instances if patient desires conservation of fertility. (Hysterectomy is Rx of choice)

VAGINAL OR VULVAR INTRAEPITHELIAL NEOPLASIA (VAIN/VIN)

Vaginal or vulvar intraepithelial neoplasia, dysplasia of the vulvovagina, and papillomatosis are often noted on vaginal/vulvar cytology prior to and after hysterectomies. Although many sources are now recommending discontinuance of Pap smears after hysterectomy, this is empirically continued at least once every 3 years secondary to the continued findings of this vaginal pathology in our area

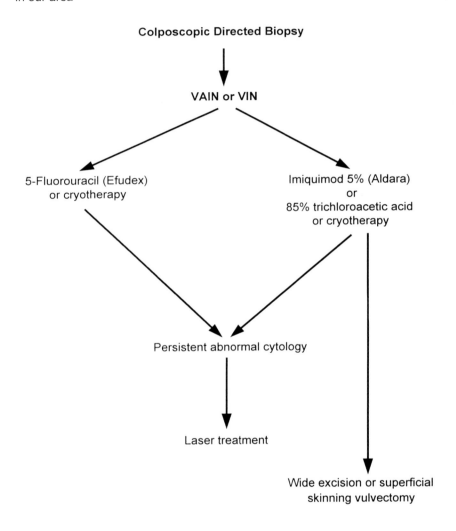

Colposcopic Directed Biopsy

VAIN or VIN

5-Fluorouracil (Efudex)
or cryotherapy

Imiquimod 5% (Aldara)
or
85% trichloroacetic acid
or cryotherapy

Persistent abnormal cytology

Laser treatment

Wide excision or superficial
skinning vulvectomy

VAGINAL OR VULVAR INTRAEPITHELIAL NEOPLASIA
(VAIN/VIN)

APPLICATION INSTRUCTIONS FOR EFUDEX (5-FU)

(1) Apply 5-FU periodically

(2) Place applicator 1/3 filled with cream (approximately 1.5 grams) deeply into the vagina

(3) Provided there is no significant inflammation or severe pain, the cream should be re-applied every 3 to 4 days

(4) You should make an appointment after 4 to 6 weeks of therapy to evaluate treatment response and side-effects. At that time if you have no significant response to therapy or if you have severe side-effects of this therapy then you might be selected for other treatments. If you have partial response you might be advised to continue the therapy for 10 full weeks. If you have complete response to therapy then you will remain under close recheck for 3 to 6 months.

Please see the informed consent and instructions that are highlighted in yellow. Please consult with me and ask me questions. After you fully understand the purpose of 5-FU and possible complications and alternatives, sign the informed consent and I will forward you a prescription.

If you have any further questions regarding this therapy, please feel free to call.

Sincerely,

John E. Turrentine, M.D.

JET/mh

This and the following page can be used for patient information and education, and as informed consent samples

VAGINAL OR VULVAR INTRAEPITHELIAL NEOPLASIA

INFORMED CONSENT AND INSTRUCTIONS FOR 5-FLUOROURACIL CREAM

You have been given a prescription for 5-fluorouracil (5-FU, Efudex) cream for the treatment of lesions on your vagina, and/or cervix. 5-FU has been used for more than 25 years in treatment of various lesions or growths of the skin. However, this medication has not been approved by the Food and Drug Administration (FDA) for use in treating warts or other precancerous growths on the genitals. A number of studies have proven the effectiveness of this drug in treating warts and "dysplasias" or abnormal growths from the wart virus. One of the major concerns using the drug is its effect on pregnancy. It is therefore vital that you are not pregnant while you are using 5-FU cream because its safety for the developing fetus is unknown. You should use close to perfect birth control (birth control pills, sterilization, abstinence, IUD, or condoms **and** diaphragm together).

Side-effects of this medication are mainly vaginal or vulvar irritation or burning which may be significant enough to stop treatment temporarily. If you notice this happening, please call the office for further instructions.

INSTRUCTIONS FOR VAGINAL USE

(1)   Use only the specially marked applicator that has been given to you or the prefilled applicators
(2)   If you do not have the prefilled applicators, please fill your applicator to the 2.0-gram mark. Double check this for the correct level
(3)   Put the applicator with the cream high into your vagina and push the plunger in
(4)   Take the applicator apart and wash with warm soapy water or throw away the prefilled applicator container
(5)   Go to bed
(6)   In the morning, get into a tub of warm water and wash out the vagina as well as you can with your fingers
(7)   You should not have intercourse for 24 hours after each cream dose
(8)   You should repeat this procedure using one dose every week for a total of 10 doses or 10 weeks

INSTRUCTION FOR VULVAR OR EXTERNAL USE

(1)   Dab a small amount (size of pea or bean) of cream onto the entire vulva while looking into a mirror. This would be best done at bedtime. Rub the white cream entirely into the vulvar skin until the cream disappears. Leave no patches of cream on the skin. Check again with a mirror
(2)   Repeat this procedure two times a week for 10 weeks
(3)   The morning after the treatment, sit in a tub of warm water and wash off any remaining cream

After either the vaginal or vulvar use, you should make an appointment for a repeat colposcopy 6 to 8 weeks after completing your last dose. If you have any questions, please call.

INFORMED CONSENT

I understand that the medication 5-FU has been prescribed for me to treat condyloma (warts) or skin changes believed to be from the wart virus. I understand that the FDA has not approved this medication for use. I also understand that it is unsafe to become pregnant while using this medication as its effects on pregnancy are unknown and that it is my responsibility to avoid pregnancy. I have had the opportunity to ask any questions I might have regarding this medication.

_____
PATIENT'S SIGNATURE

_____
DATE

_____
PROVIDER/PRACTITIONER

VERSION

EXTERNAL VERSION OF BREECH PRESENTATION OR TRANSVERSE LIE

The following patients should be excluded from consideration for external version of breech presentation:

(1)   Any patient in whom a tocolysis is contraindicated

(2)   Any patient in whom there is a high index of suspicion for utero placenta insufficiency and fetal distress

(3)   Premature labor, PROM or very dilated cervix

(4)   Multiple gestation

(5)   Third-trimester bleed, suspected abruption, placenta previa

(6)   Gestational age less than 36 weeks or estimated fetal weight greater than 3800 g

(7)   Previous uterine surgery

PROTOCOL

(1)   The risk/benefit should be discussed with the patient in advance. The patient should be aware of the risk of transient fetal bradycardia during the procedure and the occasional (less than 5%) need for urgent Cesarean. A routine hospital consent form will be signed at time of version

(2)   The patient's prenatal records, including lab work should be in Labor & Delivery

(3)   The Labor & Delivery staff and the OB Anesthesia staff should be notified of the date and time of the attempted version, and enough staff should be available at the time of the version, if a Cesarean becomes necessary

(4)   The patient should be NPO after midnight

(5)   On arrival to Labor & Delivery, a sonogram should be performed to determine:

    (a)   Fetal position and type of breech

    (b)   Estimated fetal weight

    (c)   Head extension and nuchal cord if possible

    (d)   Anomalies if possible

    (e)   Placenta location

    (f)   Amniotic fluid volume

If contraindications to version are determined the procedure should be canceled

(6)   A non-stress test should be performed and evaluated prior to the procedure

(7)   A deep-vein open IV should be inserted and a type and hold drawn

(8)   A tocolysis (terbutaline or $MgSO_4$) may be started at the lowest dose, as per protocol (see individual tocolysis protocols). Tocolysis may not be necessary in some patients

(9)   The version should be attempted as soon as the tocolytic is effective if infusion. This may be 5 minutes for subcutaneous terbutaline or 30 minutes for $MgSO_4$

(10)   The version should be done with an assistant who can provide intermittent fetal heart rate monitoring and sonograph during the procedure

(11)   After the attempted version, continue fetal monitoring for 1 hour. The patient needs a reactive NST prior to discharge

(12)   If the patient is Rh negative, a Kleihauer–Betke test should be drawn and the appropriate RhoGAM should be administered prior to discharge

VIRAL TERATOGENS

SYPHILIS

Cause:	*Treponema pallidum*
Screen:	RPR or VDRL; if + -- FTS -ABS
Infant:	Rhinitis, CNS abnormalities, deafness, mulberry molars
Treatment:	Benzathine PCN G 2.4 million units
	Test monthly RPR less than 4-fold

TOXOPLASMOSIS

Cause:	*Toxoplasma gondii* (intracellular parasite) oocysts in cat guts
Screen:	Tox IgM in Central Europe; not standard in US
Infant:	Hydrops; brain necrosis with Ca^+ deposits of ventricles; chorioretinitis; myocarditis
Treatment:	Spiramycin (1 g q. 8 hrs) and pyrimethamine (25 mg/d) if fetal infection confirmed
Prevention:	(1) Avoid eating undercooked meat; (2) wash hands after handling cat; (3) have someone else change kitty litter; (4) do not permit indoor cats to go outside; (5) do not allow stray cats in the house; (6) do not feed raw meat to cats

CYTOMEGALOVIRUS

Cause:	CMV including varicella-zoster, herpes simplex, Epstein–Barr
Screen:	None (CMV antibody in high-risk such as Day Care etc. rec by some)
Infant:	Sensorineural hearing loss, MR, chorioretinitis, deafness
Treatment:	None available. Dev of vaccine in progress
Prevention	Careful hygiene to minimize contact with toddler's saliva/urine

VARICELLA (Chicken pox)

Cause:	V-Z (respiratory droplets)
Screen.	None. 90% + (seropositive), seronegative pts exposed can be given VZIG
Infant:	Limb hypoplasia; CNS involvement; skin scarring
Treatment:	Acyclovir (neither acyclovir or VZIG dec risks of congenital malformations). No cure

RUBELLA (German measles)

Cause:	RNA virus in togavirus family (respiratory droplets or contacts)
Screen:	Rubella antibody
Infant:	Congenital heart disease; cataracts; deafness, MR
Treatment:	None
Prevention:	Rubella vaccine >90 days prior to conception or postpartum

HERPES SIMPLEX

Cause:	HSV – DNA virus – Direct intimate contact
Screen:	None
Infant:	Sp AG, PTD, IUGR. Cutaneous lesions w/in 24–48 hrs
Treatment:	Acyclovir 200 mg x 5/d or 400 mg t.i.d.
Prevention:	Acyclovir 400 mg b.i.d. in pts w/ frequent recurrences. C-section if active lesion present. (See Herpes protocol)

HIV

Cause:	Type 1 most common HIV; Low CD4+ helper T lymphocytes
Screen:	ELISA x2 – if both + – Western blot test
Infant:	No syndrome reported
Treatment:	AZT, but no cure (see Zidovudine)

PARVOVIRUS B-19/FIFTH'S DISEASE

Cause:	Parvovirus B-19 – single-stranded DNA virus
Screen	Parvovirus B-19 IgM (low Hct 2–3 wks after exposure; 2nd degree aplasia)
Infant:	Fetal hydrops; 2nd degree aplastic anemia; myocarditis; fetal hepatitis
Treatment:	None. Follow with serial ultrasounds

VULVOVAGINITIS

SYMPTOMATOLOGY

Vulvar/vaginal burning, discharge

EVALUATE VAGINA

Inspect external genitalia (r/o excoriations, blisters, ulcerations erythema, edema, atrophy)

Examine vaginal discharge – gross and microscopic

pH level –   >4.5 (bacterial vaginosis <u>OR</u> trichomoniasis)
<4.5 (physiologic <u>OR</u> uncomplicated candidal vaginitis)

Whiff test: +fishy odor =amines = anaerobic bacteria
(10% KOH) –fishy odor = normal flora
Rule out allergic/chemical irritation – careful history

CANDIDAL VAGINITIS

Part of normal vaginal flora
Risk factors:
Recent Abx, diabetes (2 hr GCT – 75 g), immunosuppression (HIV)
Diagnosis:
History – Pruritus, burning (worsened w/ urination/sexual activity)
Physical exam – Nonmalodorous, thick, white 'cottage cheese' discharge; vagina
hyperemic/edematous
Diagnostic tests   – p H = <4.5 (normal)
– microscopic – hyphal forms/budding yeast
Treatment:
Topical (first line) – terconazole, butoconazole, clotrimazole, miconazole, tioconazole
Oral (second line) – fluconazole 150 mg (not in pregnancy)

Resistant vulvovaginal candidiasis (RVVC)
(1)   Fluconazole 100 mg p.o. q. wk x6 months
(2)   Boric acid capsules 600 mg per vagina q.d. x14 days

BACTERIAL VAGINOSIS

History:	Pruritus burning, malodorous discharge (worsened during menses/after intercourse)
Physical exam:	Discharge, malodorous, thin, grey, homogenous
Diagnostic tests:	(1) pH >4.5
	(2) +Whiff test (3 out of 4)
	(3) Clue cells
	(4) Homogenous discharge
Treatment:	
Topical	– 0.75% metronidazole gel, intravaginally b.i.d. x5 days
	– 2% clindamycin cream, intravaginally q.d. x7days
Oral	– metronidazole 500 mg b.i.d. x7 days (or 250 mg t.i.d. x7 days)
	– clindamycin 300 mg b.i.d. x7 days

TRICHOMONAS VAGINALIS

History: Discharge (copious, yellow-green, homogenous, malodorous), vulvovaginal irritation, dysuria

Physical exam: Frothy, malodorous discharge, "strawberry cervix"

Diagnostic tests: pH >4.5, wet mount (mobile, flagellated organisms), trichomonads on Pap

Treatment: Oral metronidazole – 2 g p.o. x1 dose; 500 mg b.i.d. x7 days

Resistant trichomoniasis

Combination oral/vaginal metronidazole
Culture for resistant strains
Confirm treatment of partner
IV metronidazole (requires hospitalization)

ATROPHIC VAGINITIS

Thinning of vaginal epithelium, loss of rugae, friable

Treatment: Oral – 0.625 mg conjugated estrogens q. day
Topical – estrogen cream 2–4 g q.d. x2 wks and then q.o.d. x2 wks
Maintenance: estrogen 1–3x wk

TREATMENT FOR BACTERIAL VAGINOSIS

Agent	Brand name	Dosage
Metronidazole oral tablets	Flagyl	One 500 mg tab twice daily for 7 days **or** Four 500 mg tabs (2 g) in a single dose
Metronidazole 0.75% gel	Metrogel-Vaginal	5 g intravaginally twice daily x5 days*
Clindamycin 2% cream	Cleocin	5 g intravaginally x7 days
Clindamycin oral tablets	Cleocin HCl capsules	Two 150 mg capsules twice daily x7 days

*Some recommend that Metrogel can be used once daily at night for 5 days especially for milder infections

TREATMENT FOR UNCOMPLICATED CANDIDIASIS

Agent	Brand name	Dosage
Butoconazole 2% cream	Femstat*	5 g intravaginally x3 days
Clotrimazole 1% cream	Gyne-Lotrimin*	5 g intravaginally x7–14 days
	Mycelex-7	5 g intravaginally x7–14 days
Clotrimazole vaginal tabs	Gyne-Lotrimin vaginal inserts*	One 100 mg insert x7 days
	Mycelex-7 vaginal inserts*	One 100 mg insert x 7 days
	Mycelex-G vaginal tablets	One 500 mg tablet
Fluconazole oral tablets	Diflucan tablets	One 150 mg tablet
Miconazole 2% cream	Monistat 7*	5 g intravaginally for 7 days
Miconazole suppositories	Monistat 7*	One 100 mg suppository x7 days
	Monistat 3	One 200 mg suppository x3 days
Terconazole 0.4% cream	Terazol 7	5 g intravaginally x7 days
Terconazole 0.8% cream	Terazol 3	5 g intravaginally x3 days
Terconazole suppositories	Terazol 3	One 80 mg suppository x3 days
Tioconazole 6.5% vaginal	Vagistat-1	5 g intravaginally once

*Available without prescription

VULVOVAGINITIS

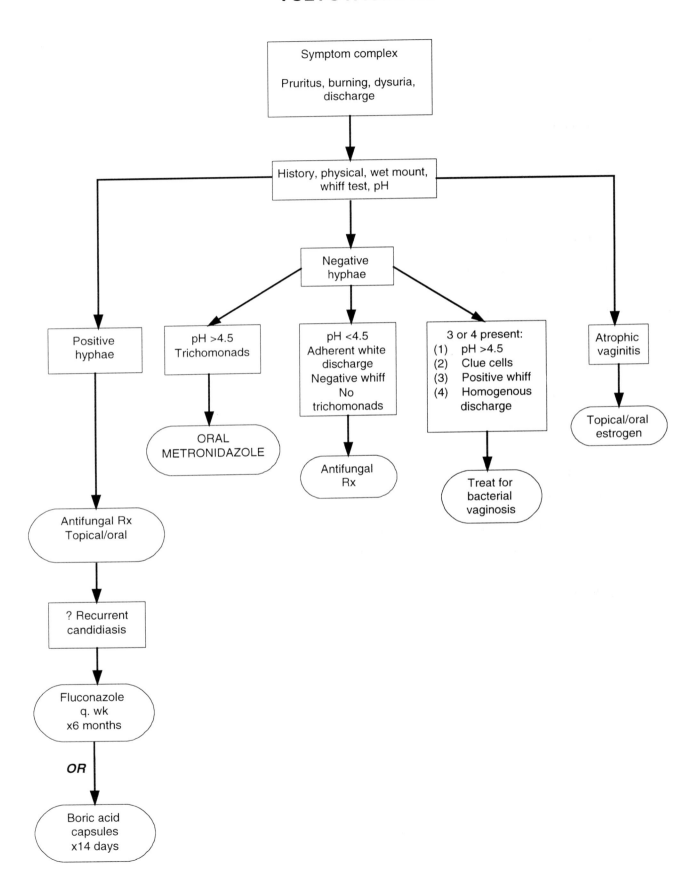

ZIDOVUDINE (AZT)

ADMINISTRATION IN PREGNANCY

Two-thirds relative reduction in vertical transmission (control 26%, treatment group 8% transmission)

Transient neonatal anemia noted in some study subjects

Consider treatment for all HIV-positive pregnant women after 14 wks EGA

All patients to receive Zidovudine should be counseled regarding benefits/risks above

ANTEPARTUM THERAPY

Zidovudine 100 mg p.o. 5x/day

INTRAPARTUM THERAPY

Recommended for any woman in pre-term labor requiring IV tocolytics and those scheduled for elective
C-section

Loading dose (2 mg/kg)

Zidovudine _____ mg in 50 ml 5% dextrose in water. Administer over 60 minutes, *or*
Zidovudine _____ mg in 50 ml 1.0% NaCl. Administer over 60 minutes

Maintenance infusion

Zidovudine 500 mg or 250 ml D5W. Rate: _____ mg/hr
or
Zidovudine 500 mg or 250 ml 0.9% NaCl. Rate: _____ mg/hr

Zidovudine ` `is stable in both NS and D5W

Choice of diluent dependent on patient needs (e.g. diabetic)

No data on IV compatibility of Zidovudine, therefore, requires separate IV line for infusion

ZIDOVUDINE

The concentration of the maintenance solution is 2 mg/ml. To calculate the rate for the infusion, divide the patient's weight (in kg) by two and round the nearest whole number. Infuse at this rate until the patient delivers. Alternatively, the chart below can be used:

Patient's weight	Rate
50 kg	25 ml/hr
52 kg	26 ml/hr
54 kg	27 ml/hr
56 kg	28 ml/hr
58 kg	29 ml/hr
60 kg	30 ml/hr
62 kg	31 ml/hr
64 kg	32 ml/hr
66 kg	33 ml/hr
68 kg	34 ml/hr
70 kg	35 ml/hr
72 kg	36 ml/hr
74 kg	37 ml/hr
76 kg	38 ml/hr
78 kg	39 ml/hr
80 kg	40 ml/hr
82 kg	41 ml/hr
84 kg	42 ml/hr
86 kg	43 ml/hr
88 kg	44 ml/hr
90 kg	45 ml/hr
92 kg	46 ml/hr
94 kg	47 ml/hr
96 kg	48 ml/hr
98 kg	49 ml/hr
100 kg	50 ml/hr